Ethics in Anaesthesia and Intensive Care

Heather Draper BA MA PhD
Senior Lecturer in Biomedical Ethics
Centre for Biomedical Ethics
Department of Primary Care
The University of Birmingham Medical School
Birmingham, United Kingdom

Wendy E Scott FRCA
Consultant Anaesthetist
Critical Care Directorate
Department of Anaesthesia
Derby City General Hospital
Derby, United Kingdom

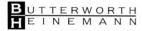

BUTTERWORTH
HEINEMANN

An imprint of Elsevier Limited

Edinburgh London New York Oxford Philadelphia St Louis Sydney Toronto 2003

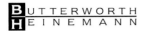

An imprint of Elsevier Limited

© 2003, Elsevier Limited. All rights reserved.

The right of Heather Draper and Wendy Scott to be identified as authors of this work has been asserted by them in accordance with the Copyright, Designs and Patents Act 1988.

First published 2003
  Reprinted 2004

ISBN 0 7506 5353 1

British Library Cataloguing in Publication Data
A catalogue record for this book is available from the British Library

Library of Congress Cataloging in Publication Data
A catalog record for this book is available from the Library of Congress

Note
Medical knowledge is constantly changing. Standard safety precautions must be followed, but as new research and clinical experience broaden our knowledge, changes in treatment and drug therapy may become necessary or appropriate. Readers are advised to check the most current product information provided by the manufacturer of each drug to be administered to verify the recommended dose, the method and duration of administration, and contraindications. It is the responsibility of the practitioner, relying on experience and knowledge of the patient, to determine dosages and the best treatment for each individual patient. Neither the Publisher nor the editors and assumes any liability for any injury and/or damage to persons or property arising from this publication.

The Publisher

 your source for books,
journals and multimedia
in the health sciences

www.elsevierhealth.com

The
publisher's
policy is to use
paper manufactured
from sustainable forests

Printed in China

Contents

Foreword

Ethics is the philosophical study of the moral value of human conduct, and of the rules and principles that ought to govern it. Where applied to a particular group, profession or individual, ethics is the code of behaviour considered to be correct. The last decade of the 20th century was remarkable for the stark relief into which the behaviour and practice of the medical and paramedical professions was thrown, following a series of high profile incidents of perceived sub-optimal care. Many aspects of the ethical framework in which medicine was practised had been taken for granted and were, to a large extent, sparingly taught and considered. At the same time the paternalistic approach of doctors to patients was increasingly becoming a thing of the past as the century ended. Patients were better informed and doctors recognised the need for informed, intelligent and sensible debate on issues of medical management from conception to death. An evolution was taking place. Suddenly the whole subject was thrown into the open and to the public scrutiny and vigorous debate.

Ethics in Anaesthesia and Intensive Care has arrived at an appropriate time. There are many troublesome issues besetting the professional lives of anaesthetists and intensivists that need to be set out and the case for present accepted practice clearly argued. In this book the authors have accepted that challenge and grasped the opportunity of setting forth the facts as presently understood, discussing the arguments and suggesting the principles through which ethical questions may be addressed. The reader may not find all the answers or indeed agree with those given, but the material is there to prepare them for the awkward and testing dilemmas that can and do arise. It is not the perrogative of any one group of people to purport to have all the answers to any ethical problems posed. Some subjects are appropriately dealt with by comprehensive reviews, while others use the combination of opinion from doctors and ethicists to facilitate the consideration of difficult subjects from more than one viewpoint. This highlights that many areas of agreement do exist, but also shows that in many areas the discussion is still not conclusive. Where a dogmatic conclusion is impossible the debate will continue. The authors have aired necessary topics, laid down positions and provided a reference point for the beginning of the 21st century. This book will assist not only anaesthetists and intensivists, but all other doctors and health care workers to consider and understand the issues, to take them forward, and to allow easier discussion for the benefit of the whole healthcare team, especially for patients and their relatives.

The complexity of many management issues in intensive care, from the use of scarce resources to an attempted definition of death, will continue to confront the original thinkers in medicine. By committing their ideas to open debate, the authors give evidence of their sensitivity and profound thought.

The book is comprehensive and is compelling reading, it will be advantageous to trainees and consultants alike, and will give a good foundation to approach many inevitable problems. It will help to formulate difficult concepts as well as rectifying erroneous beliefs or prejudices. Ideas will change as society changes, but the principles set out in this text will serve as a useful tool long into the 21st century.

S Morrell Lyons OBE MD BSC FRCA FCARCSI
Past President, Association of Anaesthetists of Great Britain and Ireland
Belfast, 2003

Acknowledgements

Our thanks go to all of those who contributed to this collection, and offer particular thanks to those who wrote at very short notice to tight deadlines. We must also thank Belinda Henry, for it is fair to say that without her gentle agitation, persistence, diplomacy and encouragement this book really would not have finally come together.

Contributors

Alan Aitkenhead BSc MBChB FRCA
Professor of Anaesthesia
Department of Anaesthesia
Queen's Medical Centre
University of Nottingham
Nottingham, UK

Chris Barham MBBS FRCA
Consultant Anaesthetist
Department of Anaesthesia
The Queen Victoria Hospital NHS Trust
East Grinstead, UK

Rebecca Bennett BA (Hons) PhD
Lecturer in Bioethics
Centre for Social Ethics and Policy
Faculty of Law
University of Manchester
Manchester, UK

Heather Draper BA MA PhD
Senior Lecturer in Biomedical Ethics
Centre for Biomedical Ethics
Department of Primary Care
The University of Birmingham
Birmingham, UK

Andrew Fagan BSc (Hons) MA
Teaching Fellow in Human Rights
Department of Philosophy
University of Essex
Colchester, UK

Lucy Frith BA (Hons) M Phil
Lecturer in Health Care Ethics
Department of Primary Care
University of Liverpool
Liverpool, UK

Catherine Hale LLB (Hons) MSc PGCE
Lecturer in Biomedical Law and Ethics
Centre for Biomedical Ethics
Department of Primary Care
The University of Birmingham
Birmingham, UK

Michael Harmer MD FRCA
Professor of Anaesthesia
Department of Anaesthesia
University of Wales College of Medicine
Cardiff, UK

David Hatch MB FRCA
Emeritus Professor of Paediatric Anaesthesia
Institute of Child Health
University of London
London, UK

June Jones MSc RGN
Lecturer in Biomedical Ethics
Centre of Biomedical Ethics
Department of Primary Care
University of Birmingham
Birmingham, UK

David Lamb BA PhD
Honorary Reader in Bioethics
Unit for Bioethics and Biomedical Science
University of Birmingham
Birmingham, UK

Richard Nicholson MA BM DCH
Editor, Bulletin of Medical Ethics
London, UK

Nicholas Pace MBChB FRCA
MRCP M Phil
Consultant Anaesthetist and
    Honorary Senior Lecturer
Department of Anaesthesia
Western Infirmary
Glasgow, UK

Lisa Schwartz BA MA PhD
Professor of Health Care Ethics
Department of Clinical Epidemiology
    and Biostatistics
McMaster University
Hamilton, Ontario
Canada

Wendy E Scott FRCA
Consultant Anaesthetist
Critical Care Directorate
Department of Anaesthesia
Derby City General Hospital
Derby, UK

Tom Sorell BA BPhil DPhil
Professor of Philosophy
Department of Philosophy
University of Essex
Colchester, UK

Richard Wenstone MBChB FRCA
Consultant in Intensive Care and
    Anaesthesia
Royal Liverpool and Broadgreen
    University Hospital
Liverpool, UK

Introduction

Heather Draper

Why have an ethics book focused on anaesthetics and intensive care; why not refer anaesthetists to a general collection on medical ethics? Indeed, why refer readers to a collection on medical ethics at all; why not just send them straight to some text on ethical theory or moral philosophy? Medical ethics is now a clearly established academic discipline and one that many practitioners from all specialties have found useful in their practical work and interesting intellectually. In the same way that moral philosophers turned their attention to the particular issues and tensions in medical (or health care) practice, so biomedical ethicists recognise that different medical specialties are facing different forms of dilemma and multilemma, and they are, in turn, responding to requests to address general medical ethics concepts to more specific problems faced by individual specialties. All those who have contributed to this collection are focusing on the concerns of anaesthetists and intensivists. It is clear that some of the specific issues raised by authors in this collection are not ones that anaesthetists share with other practitioners, or, if there are issues in common, these need to be addressed in such a way that takes into account the particular constraints on anaesthetists.

The most obvious of these specific issues is the complex working relationships that anaesthetists need to forge with other practitioners. Anaesthetists are rightly confident that they are medical specialists in their own right, and not technicians directed by surgeons, physicians, obstetricians, midwives, nurses or managers. Anaesthetists bear as much responsibility for their judgements and practice as other doctors. It would be easy for the uninitiated to think that anaesthetists and forensic pathologists have a lot in common, in that their patients are both unconscious and uncommunicative. It is certainly the case that anaesthetists do have to work with patients who are unconscious (although very many procedures are now performed under local or region blocks where the patient is awake), but this fact itself raises ethical problems. Unlike the pathologist's, anaesthetists' patients will regain consciousness and have lives to live that can be more or less affected by the decisions made by the anaesthetists who guarded their interests during a critical period of unconsciousness. But this characterisation overlooks many other aspects of anaesthetic practice. It is clear from this collection that anaesthetists do interact with patients, and they have to develop specialised skills to capitalise on what can be very short, intense and difficult circumstances in which to forge a doctor/patient relationship. Moreover, they have to develop skills as team players and negotiators to a degree that is not *required* of other specialists (however desirable these skills are in their own right). This fact is recognised over and again in the chapters that follow. The complexities of achieving mutually respectful interdisciplinary communication and joint decision making is tackled explicitly by June Jones in the context of intensive care (Chapter 12), but other authors allude to these difficulties in different contexts. This is a recurring theme in the book.

Wendy Scott and I were involved in another collection on ethics and anaesthetics that was published in 1994[1]. We have both been struck by the changes in the intervening period. There have been some quite shocking events, such as the scandals related to retained organs (and it should not be forgotten that it was an anaesthetist who blew the whistle at Bristol that led to these events unfurling), the evil and incompetence of doctors such as Harold Shipman, Rodney Ledward and Richard Neale, and the ethically dubious paediatric clinical research in Staffordshire. These events have allegedly shaken public confidence in doctors (though they have not had the noticeable effect on the demand for medical services that, for instance, the events of 11 September 2001 did on the airline industry). The General Medical Council (GMC) have responded to these kinds of high profile deficiency by setting high minimal standards for clinical practice[2] that have ethical as well as clinical competence at their core. David Hatch writes about these changes (Chapter 3). He warns us, however, that society and the profession has to think quite radically about a how to make the practice of medicine safer for patients. He argues for a system that accepts that mistakes happen which are not due solely to incompetence, and that, like the safety systems deployed by the airline industry, has checks and balances that accommodate human error.

Another major change since 1994 is the extent to which ethics has become integrated into mainstream medical practice. For qualified doctors and medical students alike, a career based partly, or even solely, in clinical ethics is both a conceivable and realistic possibility. The standard of debate on ethical matters amongst practitioners in general (and not just those with a particular interest) has increased enormously. Evidence of this is the increasing sophistication of the guidelines produced by professional bodies (like the Royal Societies, GMC and British Medical Association (BMA)). The language and detail of these documents suggests that, as a matter of routine, ordinary practitioners are equipped, willing and able to engage in conceptual debate and make finely tuned judgements rather than simply revising bullet points or applying protocols. My own chapter in this collection (Chapter 13), which revisits the familiar problem of withdrawing/withholding of treatment and euthanasia, draws enthusiastically on the BMA's lengthy document on the subject (though I do not endorse all of the BMA's arguments or conclusions). It is not uncommon for practitioners to spend time debating the ethical dimension of an individual patient's care. Ethicists are viewed more as useful partners than as a mischievous or malevolent threat, and their advisory role on professional bodies is now almost taken for granted. Medical ethics is certainly no longer an occupation for and of a minority.

The public are also being encouraged to shape the future of ethics in medicine. There have been an increasing number of public consultations on matters such as access to genetic information, pre-implantation genetic testing, anonymity of sperm donors, retained tissue, sex-selection, health protection and so on. Indeed, as a result of a very recent consultation process on the ethics and law relating to tissue donation, this collection has been unable to make any comment on the law relating to organ donation, for this is certainly going to undergo radical revision. David Lamb has, however, returned to the continuing controversy and scepticism about the reliability of tests for brainstem death and the post-mortem management of brain-dead patients who are potential organ donors (Chapter 14).

The law has changed too, subtly and explicitly. Catherine Hale is one of many authors who considers the impact of the much heralded introduction of the *Human Rights Act (1998)*, which came into force in 2000 (Chapter 4). Her review of the ethics and law of confidentiality also includes the *Data Protection Act (1998)*. She warns against the common practice of displaying patient information in intensive care units (ICUs), and reminds us of the need for vigilance in this speciality, particularly as many of the patients are unable to consent to this ready sharing of their personal information. Alan Aitkenhead's critique of consent (Chapter 2) reveals some of the more subtle changes in the law, like the modification by *Bolitho* v. *Hackney HA*[3] of the *Bolam* principle (*Bolam* v. *Friern Hospital Management Committee*[4]). Having the support of a reasonable body of medical opinion might no longer be a defence if a court decides that the opinion held by that body is itself unreasonable. We have yet to see the full effects of the *Bolitho* judgement, but it is clear that the law is also requiring doctors to have a much more heightened sense of ethics than in the past. As *Bolam* recedes as a defence against negligence, the Government, through the Department of Health, has imposed protocols for gaining consent[5]. It remains to be seen whether these protocols will promote good practice or a check-list mentality at a time when the law, the profession and the public seem to want doctors to be reflective as well as accountable.

In the wake of September 11 2001 we have all been forced to think even more carefully about how to respond to competing religious beliefs, and the place of religion in politics. The challenge posed by cultural relativism in general is address by Andrew Fagan (Chapter 5), who also explores the tension between personal belief and respect for the autonomy of others. On a less political level, differences in belief and culture pose practical problems for anaesthetists. Fagan discusses the most cited of these – the Jehovah's witness – but there are many occassions when it is difficult to reconcile what the patient believes is right with what the clinician thinks is ethically acceptable, or permissible for a clinician to do. In Nicholas Pace's chapter (Chapter 6), it quickly becomes clear that, in the case of children, it can be legitimate to balance the right of the competent child to consent for himself or herself against the right of the child to protection, and that parents and society have rights in relation to children that must also be taken into account. Moreover, clinicians have an overriding duty to act in the interests of their child patients. In this potential maelstrom of competing interests, rights and obligations, it is easy to see how we have arrived at a situation where competent children are entitled to consent to treatment (which one supposes would not have been offered if the clinician did not think it best) but children have no independent right to refuse treatment. This is one solution to the tension between autonomy and different views about best interests. As a moral philosopher, this solution seems to me to work only because the concept of legal competence does not strictly equate to the ethical notion of autonomy, and because the legal mechanism exists to impose the beliefs of adults on to children.

The ethical position in the case of the foetus is no less of a maelstrom of competing interests but, because a foetus does not have the same legal protection as a child, the interests of the pregnant woman tend to carry greater legal weight. But how are the interests of a pregnant woman to be defined? The usual assumption is that it is in her interests to have an untraumatic delivery and a healthy child (or children) as a result. There may, however, be a difference of opinion between the woman, her obstetrician or midwife, and the anaesthetist about what constitutes as an untraumatic delivery, or how best to ensure a good outcome for the baby. The ethical problems that this can generate are discussed by Wendy Scott (Chapter 10), along with other dilemmas facing obstetric anaesthetists, such how to gain valid consent to site an epidural when a woman is in extreme pain, or when she has made a previous and explicit refusal of consent.

Lisa Schwartz's discussion of the teaching of ethics and law to medical students (Chapter 16) throws a different light on the problem of tolerance to cultural and ethical differences, sometimes known as relativism. She argues that there is a danger in medical ethics teaching that students learn to be so sympathetic to the views of others that they become paralysed when it comes to making professional decisions of their own. She draws attention to the fact that a great deal is expected from ethics and law teaching in the current climate in the UK, and not all the aims are easily reconciled. Her chapter (written before the GMC produced *Tomorrows Doctors*, 2002[6] – but no less relevant for this) illustrates the problems of trying to get the various balances right in teaching. Medical schools are certainly challenging places to be in 2003. There is no less rivalry between specialities, but increased financial pressures mean that many academics are finding it difficult to keep a reasonable balance between their teaching, clinical and research commitments. Moreover, those involved with teaching face the new challenge of the introduction of four-year graduate entry programmes, many of which are wholeheartedly embracing problem-based learning for the first time, so that it is not just the content of the curriculum that is under scrutiny, but also the style of learning. More established practitioners also have to adjust to different styles of learning and demonstrating skills in order to gain re-accreditation. One of the aims of this collection is to help those preparing postgraduate qualifications, as well as, of course, providing an element of continuing education to established practitioners.

In 1994, Michael Vickers wrote: 'resources will never be sufficient to satisfy demand'. He also predicted that scoring systems were a 'ticking time bomb' and that triage would have to become acceptable in ICU, particularly in relation to 'hopeless' cases (pp. xvii–xviii[1]). Richard Wenstone's chapter (Chapter 11) graphically illustrates that anaesthetists are still facing the problem of trying to provide a service when the budget allocated cannot meet the demand for care, and they have still not – not for want of trying but because the task is almost impossible – resolved the practical and ethical difficulties of admission policies. Wenstone also subtly discusses the role and relative importance of evidence in decision-making. Lucy Frith explores the use of evidence-based medicine more explicitly and philosophically (Chapter 9). She does not doubt the need for evidence in medical decision-making, but she does put under close scrutiny the idea that there is such a thing as a 'best treatment' that can be derived from data divorced from an individual patient's values.

There has undoubtedly been increased pressure on clinicians to use evidence-based practice since the National Institute for Clinical Excellence was established in 1999. This evidence, however, has to be gathered. The UK has recently been exposed to several independent and appalling stories where the rights of individuals have been violated in the name of medical progress. Mindful of these incidents, the value and importance of research and the increasing pressure on clinicians to participate in research and audit, this collection includes two chapters on research ethics. Michael Harmer addresses the responsibilities of practitioners involved in clinical research (Chapter 7), and Richard Nicholson looks at the some of the history of attempts to regulate research in the interests of human participants, the establishment, role and function of research ethics committees (RECs), and the introduction of governance arrangements for RECs (Chapter 8). It is clear that there are many hurdles in the path of medical research. One is that the public perception about research is very mixed. On the one hand, there is concern that some researchers seem blind to patients' rights or welfare (at best because they are over-enthusiastic, or at worst because they are unscrupulous), and there is concern that some individuals are unfairly excluded from the potential benefits of research. On the other hand, there is some support for evidence-based decisions (patients often come to a consultation having already searched the internet for information on their condition and possible remedies); there is willingness to participate in research and considerable generosity to charities whose specific remit is to fund research. There is also the ever present danger that people want the benefits of research but want immunity from the associated risks, and clinical researchers, like other clinicians, may feel compelled to practice defensively. As both Harmer and Nicholson suggest, maintaining public trust and confidence is vital, and obviously the best way of achieving this is by ensuring research is as ethical as possible, both in terms of its design and methodology and in the way in which the protocols are followed and data collected and analysed. Both individual researchers and RECs have a part to play here, and they should be striving to generate a mutually reinforcing working partnership. This can only be achieved if two perceptions are confined to history. The first, and older, perception is that RECs are in the pocket of the researchers. The second is when RECs and researchers see each other, rather than unethical research, as the common enemy. There is too much at stake for either of these outdated views to persist anywhere in the research community.

One advance in medical knowledge that has the potential to change thinking in ethics and social policy is the massive improvement in the clinical management of human immunodeficiency virus (HIV) infection. The potential life-expectancy, and quality of life, of those who test positive for HIV is such that some insurance companies are now offering life insurance to people who are HIV positive. This suggests that insurers not only anticipate that such individuals will live for longer but also that they will be sufficiently healthy to earn enough income to pay the premiums. This change in prognosis has shifted the debate about testing. In the early 1990s, it was argued that the disadvantages of knowing one's HIV status far outweighed the advantages. This, along with the huge stigma attached to being HIV positive, meant that HIV was treated as a special case in public health with no provision for mandatory testing or contact tracing. As Rebecca Bennett illustrates in her chapter (Chapter 15) on testing for blood-borne communicable disease, it is now argued that HIV should not be treated as a special case but should be on a par with other blood-borne communicable infections, like hepatitis C (it is also worth noting that the GMC no longer distinguishes between HIV and other infectious diseases in its guidelines). The threat posed by HIV, however, has helped to refocus the debate about testing for infectious disease in general. HIV challenged the assumption that containment, mandatory testing, the public interest and paternalism were all acceptable principles to apply in disease control. Bennett explores the tension between the protection of individual autonomy (the 'right' not to know and the 'right' not to be tested without consent) and public health policies that mitigate in favour of routine testing in the public interest. She is also particularly concerned that pregnant women are routinely tested without being fully informed and wonders whether this suggests that routine testing in general is acceptable or that routine testing of pregnant women is actually unacceptable. She addresses this question in the context of routine testing for health-care professionals, both in their own interests and in the interests of their patients.

In the final contributions to this collection (Chapter 17), Christopher Barham and Tom Sorell look at the ethical issues raised when anaesthetists undertake private work. Barham gives a comprehensive and favourable overview of the ethical issues involved in private practice. Sorell is more cautious, arguing that there are moral risks in embracing private practice as it may be damaging both to the National Health Service (NHS) and to professional detachment. Involvement with the private sector, both in terms of encouraging two health systems (one public and one private) and in terms of public–private financial partnerships, seems to be near the top of the current political agenda. It may take another ten years for us to discover whether private medicine and private finance will save or erode the NHS. What seems regrettable is that so many doctors have come to view their private practice as an opportunity to practice, without managerial and administrative constraint, the craft they went to medical school to learn and as a means of maintaining their clinical standards.

This collection does not necessarily represent our own views and authors were not briefed on the kinds of conclusions we would like them to draw about the role of ethics in anaesthesia and intensive care, nor about how particular ethical issues should be resolved. As a result, some chapters are more argumentative than others, and some of the views expressed are controversial while others are less so. Some chapters aim to provide an overview of issues in a particular area, others are focused on just a few issues and do not pretend to be comprehensive. Some chapters include a response, but this does not indicate that the first author has offered particularly controversial views. Rather, we were fortunate that additional authors were willing to add their views to those that had already been expressed.

The second section of this introduction is a reworking of the first chapter of the Scott, Vickers and Draper collection[1]. It has been modified to suit its new surroundings, and it was included because it was felt (by one of us) that readers would appreciate a steer in the theory direction. The rest of the collection will be accessible to those who want to start addressing the issues in practice without reading on here!

Ethical theory

One way of understanding ethical theory is to work from an example. In the context of this book, a good example to work from is one in which the death of a patient occurs.

Being a subject of moral concern

The first thing to note is that a subject has been identified and that this subject – the patient – is assumed to be worthy of moral consideration. Briefly, a being is considered to be worthy of moral consideration if that being exhibits such characteristics as an ability to suffer (a formulation which would include all sentient life), or rationality (one which might exclude some or all animals and some human beings). By this standard, pebbles, for instance, are not objects worthy of moral consideration. In the case of abortion, on the other hand, arguments about the status of the foetus are often made in response to assumptions that the foetus either is, or is not, worthy of moral consideration; that the foetus is, or is not, the kind of being that can be wronged. Similar arguments surround the question of whether a patient in a persistent/permanent vegetative state (PVS) can be wronged by the withdrawal of therapy. One way in which relatives might address this question is by saying the person they loved died a long time ago, indicating that the dead (in this case loosely speaking) do not command the same moral respect as the living.

Being a moral agent or having moral responsibility

The next thing to note in the example of the death of a patient is that someone is assumed to have caused the death, someone who is responsible for his or her actions, someone who can be praised or blamed and held accountable for these actions. To be considered a morally responsible agent, one must be autonomous, at least in the sense that one is competent and acting voluntarily. In this sense of responsibility, a mouse cannot be held responsible for causing a death by chewing through a power cable to an intensive care unit, nor can a young child who innocently unplugs a life support machine. The identification of the moral agent is important because it is one of the factors that distinguishes accidents from moral incidents. Also, it is generally through a consideration of the responsibilities of the identified agent that ethical issues are discussed, for example, who should have done (or not done) X, and who had the duty to do X. In healthcare ethics, the agent is usually assumed to be a health-care professional. However, in some cases, the ethical debate itself may be over the correct identification of the moral agent. For instance, where a doctor withdraws therapy at the insistence of a patient, some may wish to argue that if the patient was competent and so forth (i.e. an autonomous agent) and refused treatment then the patient was responsible for his/her own death. Others might hold that since it was the doctor who performed the action, the doctor must be held accountable for the consequences. Under other circumstances it may be inappropriate to identify one person as the agent responsible, perhaps because the decision was made by a team of people. This does not mean that no one is responsible for team decisions: all members of a team may be jointly responsible. On the other hand, perhaps team decisions, as such, are never made. Perhaps one person decides having canvassed the views of others.

The significance of consequences, intentions and motives

The description of the situation of the agent and the patient also matters. When a patient dies, we want to know more about the situation than simply that the patient died. The cases in which there is ethical interest are those where an agent causes the patient's death through an act or an omission. However, two identical actions or omissions can have very different outcomes, so part of the description of what happened must include the consequences. An injection that results in a patient's death is more serious than one that does not. Or is it? If I intend that an injection should kill a patient but I miscalculate the dose required and the patient does not die, there might be a legal difference (i.e. attempted murder rather than murder) but is there a significant moral difference? Some people believe that acting upon an intention to kill someone is equally bad whether or not one is successful. Others might reserve judgement until they know why I was trying to kill my patient, thereby placing an emphasis on motive. My good motives (of wanting to relieve suffering) might incline them to identify the killing as euthanasia (which they may believe to be acceptable) rather than murder (which is wrong by definition).

The distinction between justified killing and murder does not only depend upon motives: it might also be related to consequences. Here the focus of attention is not so much on what happens, but what results and how these results compare with the other possible outcomes of the other available actions. Thus, an outcome which puts an end to suffering might be preferred to one in which the patient's suffering is prolonged, and it is the outcome (the relief of suffering) rather than the means by which it is achieved (the killing) which is the decisive factor.

Irrespective of where the emphasis should lie in the description of what occurs, it is important also to recognise that the agent must, either by an act or failure to act, cause the consequences. This emphasis on cause is central to one of the contemporary ethical preoccupations in intensive care, namely, how futility is to be defined. If a patient will die whatever one does, it would be seriously unjust to hold the doctor responsible for events that are effectively beyond the doctor's control or influence. Whilst, however, it is possible to be causally but not morally responsible for something (an accident for instance), causal responsibility is a pre-requisite for moral responsibility. In short, causal responsibility is a necessary but not sufficient component of moral responsibility.

Moral theories

Virtue theory concerns itself with the character and qualities of the agent. Other theories focus on the action itself, or what was intended by the action. This latter kind of theory generates rules governing actions, which are absolutes such as 'it is wrong to kill under any circumstances'. Such theories are known as deontological theories (from the Greek *deon*, meaning duty). Theories that concentrate solely on the outcome of actions are called consequentialist. What distinguishes consequentialist theories from each other is their perspective on what makes a consequence good or bad. Deontological theories and consequential theories have more in common with each other than either has with virtue theory. Although their answers are different, deontologists and consequentialists are both addressing the question 'what should I do?' Virtue theory, because it is centred on the human agent, is more concerned with the question 'what kind of person should I be?'

When practitioners discuss an ethical issue in healthcare, they often implicitly appeal to one (or more) of these theoretical approaches. For instance, a statement such as 'whenever I have to make a hard decision, I try to think like the first consultant I ever worked for. He was such good man, respected by patients and colleagues alike because he always exercised excellent judgement' draws on virtue theory. Whereas the statement 'respecting confidentiality is important; patients tell us things in belief that we will keep what they say secret; breaching confidentiality is wrong because it's breaking a kind of promise' is an example of deontological reasoning. And the statement 'if I treat this patient, a bed will be blocked for many months that could be used to treat several other patients: it's as simple as that' is a consequentialist justification. There is no definitive answer as to which of these theories is the best or right one to use. Whilst we might identify more closely with one theory rather than another, examples can be found which weaken our commitment to a single method of resolving our moral problems. This does not necessarily mean that it is pointless to explore such theories because, in so doing, we can often isolate the source of our concerns about some decision, have a greater insight into our decision making, and a greater understanding of the moral principles that underpin our actions. We may also learn to argue more consistently.

Virtue theory   Virtue is a disposition to be good. A virtuous person is one whose character is consistently good in all departments of life. Different circumstances and different roles might require the exercise of different virtues. Virtuous doctors might be impartial as far as patients are concerned, but totally partial when dealing with their own families. One's virtue cannot, therefore, be assessed just by looking down a list of one's actions, just as one cannot identify someone as a liar on the basis of one lie. Being a liar is a character trait that one might expect to manifest itself in all aspects of life, and being an honest person is consistent with being less than truthful on occassions.

One way of identifying virtue is by contrasting it with vice. Aristotle claimed that virtue is the golden mean between two contrasting vices. Courage, for instance, is the mean between recklessness and cowardice. By mean, he does not intend some kind of halfway point, but rather a value that changes according to inclination and circumstance. Under some circumstances, courage might require one to act more recklessly than at other times; sometimes one has to stand and fight and at other times one should walk away and live to fight another day. This way of assessing virtues also takes into account that people are, by inclination, different, and that what for me seems to be bordering on recklessness might seem merely commonplace to you. Consequently, to be virtuous I might have to force myself to be more reckless, whilst you might have to incline yourself to be more cowardly.

Being able to recognise a virtuous person, or assess what virtue is, does not really answer the question of why one ought to aim to be virtuous in the first place. The reason given by Aristotle was that being virtuous or good was a means of being truly happy, and was, therefore, in our best interests. At this point, virtue theory begins to sound like consequentialism. As we shall see, both the consequentialist theories of utilitarianism and egoism may tell us that we should do what makes us happy. Aristotle's view of happiness is associated neither with individual preference nor sentient gratification: it has to do with flourishing as a human being. In his view, flourishing in this way is the highest good and as such requires no justification. It, of itself, justifies any means necessary to secure it. As far as Aristotle was concerned, only by exercising the virtues of courage, temperance and justice can one flourish. Moreover, flourishing is not something that one achieves totally by or for oneself; it also has to do with society. Thus, Aristotle's ideal of the virtuous man (women were not considered fully able to be virtuous because they were not considered fully rational, and neither were slaves) was someone whose energies were directed to social well-being through military or political office. Modern Aristotelianism also holds that virtue leads to flourishing and that flourishing is the highest good. However, the example for all to follow is not, as in Aristotle, a man in high office but someone who is spontaneously and consistently decent in a more everyday way. Examples of great courage are not drawn from acts of war or politics but from everyday behaviour. Hursthouse[7], for instance, uses the example of women becoming pregnant or continuing with a pregnancy in the knowledge that giving birth may be a very painful experience. Whereas Aristotle's view centred on three main virtues (justice, temperance and courage), modern virtue theory tends to lay equal emphasis on a multitude of virtues such as friendship, benevolence, patience, compassion, caring as well as justice, temperance and courage.

Virtue theory has particular relevance to health professionals, especially those whose roles have traditionally been associated with intimate care and empathy – such as nursing. Even traditional medicine, male-dominated and male-oriented with its emphasis on learning through experience in a baptism of fire, might readily associate itself with classical virtue theory: men battling against disease, under trying circumstances, manifesting courage, allocating scarce resources justly, and temperately keeping their feelings hidden in the face of great suffering. Such men made decisions and ran the health service in the same way as Aristotle's elite ran the city-states. Ironically, health care in which the patient is a passive receiver of the virtues and skills of the attendant physician highlights several of the weaknesses of Aristotle's concept of virtue. It was very elitist: basically, including only wealthy and powerful men. Also, the three central virtues tend to be emotionally very dry with an almost cold, dispassionate exercise of goodness, where the value of the subject of the virtues was merely to facilitate the virtuous behaviour of the agent. A revised Aristotelian theory could facilitate the existing shift away from this model of medicine to one where the professional and patient are in a more equal partnership of care; one where medical students are encouraged to acknowledge that watching someone die, and later telling the relatives, is personally distressing; one where more democratic teams of carers are involved; and one where it is theoretically possible for people of both sexes and all backgrounds to compete for positions of authority.

The difficulty of depending for guidance on the rules of religion is not that these rules require us to do things that would otherwise be considered wrong, although they may do. Indeed, religious rules often have a great deal in common with those Kant generated from rational principles alone. The problem lies in the justification of the rules in the light of the question 'why ought I to obey this law?' For instance, the 'thou shalt not kill' law is frequently challenged in cases of painful terminal illness or severe disability. The most obvious criticism of religious dictates is that different religions, even sects of the same religion, can have different rules, and it seems impossible to determine which has the monopoly on divine wisdom.

There is a sense in which the 'good' doctor is not just the one who is clinically competent, but one who is good in the moral sense as well. This is reflected in the current shift to problem-based medical training where students learn by integrating different kinds of knowledge and, especially relevant in terms of this book, where clinical and ethical learning is done simultaneously. Indeed, the distinction between the clinical and the ethical is largely artificial as a good clinical decision should, almost by definition, also be morally good.

Deontology   Rules governing conduct can come from a variety of sources. They can be formulated individually after careful reflection; they can be acquired from parents or society (the law and professional guidelines are good examples here); they can flow from religious belief; or they can be generated from rational principles (like the deontological theory that is the focus of this section, namely that based on Kant).

The difficulty of depending for guidance on the rules of religion is not that these rules require us to do things that would otherwise be considered wrong, although they may do. Indeed, religious rules often have a great deal in common with those Kant generated from rational principles alone. The problem lies in the justification of the rules in the light of the question 'why ought I to obey this law?' For instance, the 'thou shalt not kill' law is frequently challenged in cases of painful terminal illness or severe disability. The most obvious criticism of religious dictates is that different religions, even sects of the same religion, can have different rules, and it seems impossible to determine which has the monopoly on divine wisdom.

A more damaging criticism highlights problems inherent in appeals to divine justification. If I answer the question 'why should I obey this rule?' with 'because God dictates that I should', then two further issues need to be addressed, one following from the other. In a sense, the answer given begs the question because it does not tell me why I should do what God dictates. If I do what God dictates because I fear eternal damnation, then the reason why I obey God is because God has power over me. It is this power alone that motivates my compliance. Under threat of eternal damnation, I probably would obey the same law even if I knew that God was in fact an evil demon. The mere fact that someone has the power to impose rules does not, of itself, make these rules good. On the other hand, if I do what God dictates because I think that what God dictates is good, then I am bound to address the ancient question 'is it good because the gods command it, or do the gods command it because it is good?' If this rule is commanded by God because it is good, then this goodness is a self-sufficient reason for obeying; the fact that God endorses it too is neither here nor there (and my answer to the question posed should simply be that I am obeying this rule because it is good). If I wish to preserve God's omnipotence in moral matters and assert instead that it is a good rule because God commands it, I am back to the problem of follow-ing any rule, good or bad, simply because it is commanded by God. If I try to argue that God is by nature simply incapable of commanding something that is not good, I am then faced with the first criticism, namely determining whether what I believe has indeed been divinely commanded when the woman next door believes that she has been similarly commanded to take the opposite view.

Kant's theory, whilst yielding rules in keeping with Christian ethics, does not depend upon the existence of God for its justification. Indeed, from his point of view, following dictates of morality because of fear of divine punishment is an act of prudence: a sensible rather than moral act, an act in *accordance with* rather than *from* duty. He asserted that the only justification for acting morally is that moral action is right. Any other justification is conditional, and if the conditions imposed do not apply then there is no longer an incentive for acting. For ex-ample, if I tell my children not to tell lies or I'll punish them, they will have no reason to tell the truth when I'm not around to hear them. However, if I tell them not to tell lies because to do so is wrong, they will (hopefully) tell the truth even when I'm not in earshot. Kant was able to adopt this position because he argued that truly moral rules were also totally in accord with reason. Thus, just as two plus two will always equal four, moral rules must apply without exception: that is, unconditionally. Rather than generate his version of the Ten Commandments, he provided a test for moral action – the categorical imperative – which means just what it says. It is something that must be done (is imperative) without excep-tion (categorically). Because rules that are moral are unconditional, they must also be universal. Thus, Kant's three formulations of the categorical imperative are:

- Act only on those maxims (rules) that you can at the same time will to be universal laws (only do this thing if you are prepared for it to be done universally).
- Treat no one, including yourself, merely as a means to an end, but only and always as an end in his/herself.
- Act as though you were making laws not just for yourself but for everyone living in the kingdom of ends.

The first is straightforward, even if one disagrees with it. Part of what it says is that I should only lie or kill if I am prepared for everyone else to lie and kill too.

The examples just given show how Kant was able to claim that morality accords with reason, since, for example, it is pointless to lie to the bank manager if the bank manager assumes that everyone is lying. Thus, to will that lying becomes a universal law is self-defeating and, therefore, irrational. The second formulation has to do with Kant's notion of what it is to be a moral agent. For him, morality applied only to rational beings because only rational beings are capable of choice and, therefore, of autonomous action. It makes sense that I should only be praised or blamed for that which I did when I could have chosen not to. It would be unjust to praise or blame me for that which I was compelled to do, either by instinct or force. In this sense, instinct has to do with animal aspects of behaviour. Whilst I cannot be blamed for feeling hungry, how I choose to satisfy my hunger is open to moral evaluation. The second formulation demands respect for autonomy. This imperative also perfectly conforms to reason, since if I use someone as a means to my own ends, I must be prepared for this to be a universal law, thereby undermining my own autonomy and effectively rendering myself unable even to make this decision to use the other person. Respect for humanity complements the sorts of rules generated by the first formulation. Not only is it irrational to lie, but lying also uses the deceived as a means to the end of the deceiver. Telling the truth allows people to make up their minds for themselves. Lying is a form of manipulation that undermines the autonomy of the deceived. It is wrong on two counts: first, it treats oneself as an exception to a universal law (liars only succeed because most people tell the truth), and is thus unjust; second, it undermines the autonomy of the deceived.

The first categorical imperative also means that ethical behaviour is impartial – we have the same responsibilities whoever we are and under whatever circumstances we find ourselves. This supports the establish practice in medicine of non-judgemental treatment. At the same time, however, the duties to patients are the same as the duties we owe to ourselves. Patients should not be used as a means to the ends of doctors, and by the same token doctors should not be used as means to the ends of patients, or anyone else. Kantian ethics entitles doctors to protect themselves within the limits of due respect to the autonomy of others.

Kantianism is a controversial means of decision-making in health-care ethics. For instance, everyone agrees that doctors have a duty to care for patients and to maintain confidentiality, but few would want to hold that such duties are absolute and overriding in all circumstances. A case can always be found where adherence to some duty seems to have such negative consequences that to act upon it seems immoral rather than highly principled. It is in these cases that utilitarian concerns come to the fore. Before moving on to this theory, we should look at one further principle associated with deontology – the doctrine of double effect – which is often present in discussions about euthanasia, withdrawal of treatment and palliative care.

Double effect   This doctrine has uncharitably been described as a deontological excuse for doing something that would normally be absolutely prohibited. It is most commonly used as a way of justifying the giving of pain relief for the purpose of relieving pain, but in the knowledge that so doing shortens life. Those who question the doctrine do so on the grounds that it appears to be a case of moral alchemy – something that makes a deontologically wrong act appear to be good just when the going gets tough for the deontologist.

The doctrine makes four stipulations, all of which must apply for the doctrine to hold:

- The action, or inaction, must be morally permissible.
- Only the good and not the bad effects of what is done must be intended.
- The bad effects must not be the means by which the good effect is brought about.
- There must be proportionality between the good and bad effects.

In terms of pain relief, for example:

- The relief of pain is itself a good thing to do.
- In the giving of analgesia, the intention must only be to relieve the pain, not to bring about the patient's death.
- Death itself must not be used as a means of pain relief.
- It is unacceptable to use pain relief in the knowledge that it will hasten death if the pain is not great or if it will be relatively short lived. Therefore, occasions where such pain relief would be justified only usually occur when the patient would be likely to die soon anyway and the pain will not respond to a lesser dose or an alternative combination of drugs.

As far as the doctrine is concerned, then, there is a difference between giving pain relief that kills the patients and killing the patient to relieve the pain. Clearly, the emphasis remains firmly on what is intended rather than either precisely what is done or the outcome. This leads to two criticisms: first, what is intended cannot be divorced from what one foresees will happen; second, what matter are consequences, irrespective of intentions, so that if the outcome is good, the action that caused it must be good.

There is insufficient time to look at the doctrine in any greater depth than this, except to add that it is important to keep in mind a distinction between what, in principle, might make an action good and bad, and proving that this principle was indeed acted upon. Often, discussion about the principle of double effect degenerates into a debate about whether one could prove what the agent intended to do. The fact that the doctrine of double effect might be used to hide a bad action does not invalidate it in principle, it merely means that it is difficult to use as a reliable means of assessing all but our own intentions.

Consequentialism   The two most commonly cited consequentialist theories are egoism and utilitarianism. Egoism claims that what people should do is that which it is in their best interests to do. Indeed, some egoists hold that this is all we are capable of doing. However, there is a difference between being selfish and being self-interested. Self-interest is compatible with morality, and it may be required by morality. This is not just because one might be punished for failing to behave well. Rather, it is in our interests to be part of a society that respects life, property, truth and justice. So, the egoist might adhere to the same rules as the Kantian but for different reasons: reasons that Kant himself illustrated in his example of the honest shopkeeper. Whilst the Kantian shopkeeper will give the correct change because this is the right thing to do, the egoist will give the correct change because, in the long run, short-changing is bad for business. Egoism can give rise to what is known as social contract theory – in short, a view that we need to arrive at a set of rules that everyone can live by and which do not unduly disadvantage particular individuals or groups of individuals so that it is in the interests of us all to keep to the rules.

Utilitarianism considers that what one should aim for is the greatest good and the least harm. An action is good – and, therefore, required – if it achieves the most good and the least harm. It is the ends that count and not the means. Accordingly, killing, deceiving, promise breaking, etc. are only wrong if they fail to achieve the most good and the least harm. Nothing is absolutely wrong; it all depends upon the circumstances. This does not mean, though, that utilitarians would kill, deceive or break their promises lightly; like the egoist, they will assess consequences in the long as well as the short term. On the whole, people are happier if they are safe from killing, lying or cheating, but utilitarianism also recognises that on occasions *refraining* from killing, lying or cheating also has terrible consequences, and that avoiding such consequences has to be a function of morality.

There are many forms of utilitarianism, each with its own definition of what constitutes a good consequence: for instance, maximising happiness or individual preference or well-being or pleasure. Not only does utilitarianism have the problem of defining what is meant by good, it also has to calculate and, therefore, quantify goodness. Even if goodness, or indeed harm, could be quantified in this way, it is far from clear that objective calculations could be made since the consequences of actions are infinite, and to limit the calculation seems to be arbitrary and, therefore, unjust. Utilitarianism also claims that everyone counts and no one counts for more than one. It is arguable, therefore, that I am acting less than well if I only take into account the effects that my actions have on myself, family, colleagues or patients, even though these people matter more to me than others.

These problems notwithstanding, utilitarianism is a theory that has considerable attractions. It includes within its scope all sentient life, and it has been an inspiration for many movements against oppression and discrimination. Many utilitarian writers are associated with the development of health-care ethics because they were able to challenge traditional views, such as the view that killing is always wrong. This greatly influenced the debate about euthanasia. Likewise, utilitarianism can justify the otherwise unpalatable need to take resources from some patients in order to provide services for others. Since it is the consequences that count, utilitarianism also fits comfortably into the resource management preoccupation with 'opportunity costs' (the opportunities that are lost when money is spent in one place rather than another). Treating acts and omissions equally according to consequences also enables utilitarians to argue in favour of active euthanasia whenever a decision for passive euthanasia has been made, because to do so ensures a quick rather than lingering death. It is, therefore, perceived to be a very practical theory, addressing the circumstances as they are rather than as one would like to find them.

The problem with utilitarianism is that, as with deontology, it occasionally requires some uncomfortable decisions to be made. In utilitarianism, there is nothing wrong with killing one person to save five – even where the one is a perfectly healthy victim, who is sacrificed at random in order to provide donor organs for the dying five[8]. This is not a decision most doctors are eager to justify, but, under some circumstances, it can be desirable to sacrifice the interests of the patient for the interests of others: for instance, it is sometimes desirable to breach confidentiality. But, equally, there are occasions where it seems plainly wrong to sacrifice the interests of individuals for the greater good.

References

1. Scott W, Vickers M, Draper H. Ethical Issues in Anaesthesia. London: Butterworth-Heinmann, 1994
2. General Medical Council. Good Medical Practice. London: GMC, 1998
3. *Bolitho v. Hackney HA* [1993] 4 Med. LR 381
4. *Bolam v. Friern Hospital Management Committee* [1957] 1 WLR 582
5. Department of Health. Good practice in consent implementation guide: consent to examination or treatment. London: Department of Health, 2001
6. General Medical Council. Tomorrow's Doctors. London: GMC, 2002
7. Hursthouse R. Beginning Lives. Oxford: Blackwell, 1988
8. Harris J. The Survival Lottery. In: Applied Ethics. P Singer, ed. Oxford: Oxford University Press, 1986: 85–87

Consent and Adult Patients in Anaesthesia and Intensive Care

2

Alan Aitkenhead

Introduction

Consent is a state of mind: a decision by a patient. The competent adult patient has a fundamental right under common law to give, or to withhold, consent to examination, investigation or treatment. This is a basic principle of health care. Any treatment, investigation or physical contact with the patient undertaken without consent may amount to battery.* It is highly unlikely that a health-care professional would be charged with criminal assault for treating a patient without consent; a criminal charge would be appropriate only if harm was intended or was an obviously foreseeable risk. However, a patient who is able to demonstrate battery in a civil court is entitled to compensation for the battery itself; in addition, the patient may be able to claim compensation for any injury suffered, even when the treatment has been conducted competently. The limitation period in respect of civil claims arising from injuries caused by battery is six years, compared (usually) with three years for claims arising from medical negligence. Battery by medical practitioners is regarded by the General Medical Council as an offence that may constitute serious professional misconduct; it may also result in employers invoking disciplinary procedures.

Patients consent to treatment after receiving information about the treatment and about material risks that may be associated with the treatment. A material risk is one to which a reasonable person in the patient's position would be likely to attach significance. If a foreseeable complication materialises from a risk that was not mentioned, the patient may argue that consent for the procedure would not have been given if the risk of that complication had been explained. This has two potential consequences in law.

The patient may argue that the consent was invalid, and that performance of the procedure amounted to battery as a result of failure to obtain 'informed consent'. However, outside the United States of America, this has found little favour

---

*A battery is an unauthorised physical contact. In an assault, the victim is caused to fear that a battery is about to occur. In most medical cases in which unauthorised physical contact occurs, there is no assault.

with the Courts, which have taken the view that a charge of battery cannot be sustained provided that the patient has been advised in broad terms of the nature of the procedure to be performed.

Alternatively, the patient may argue that, by refusing to undergo the procedure if appropriate warnings had been given, the complication would have been avoided. If this argument is successful, then the patient is entitled to compensation for the consequences of the injury, even if the injury occurred despite all reasonable care in undertaking the procedure. Thus, in contrast to claims for negligent treatment, it is not necessary for the patient to show that the standard of care in performance of the procedure was inadequate; it is necessary only to demonstrate that the warnings which were given did not conform to an acceptable standard and that if the warning had been given, the patient would not have consented to undergo the procedure.

In theory, the test in law is based on a comparison between the risks that were explained and the risks that a reasonable doctor would have mentioned (see the discussion of *Sidaway* below). In clinical negligence claims that centre on the standard of clinical care and often involve very complex issues, judges rely on expert evidence to determine the standard of care that would have been regarded as appropriate by a reasonable and responsible body of medical opinion at the time. Judges have no experience in medical practice, and must base their judgements on the opinions of doctors who have experience in the relevant field. However, judges are actual or potential patients, and they are able to form their own view as to the adequacy of information provided to a patient, irrespective of evidence about the risks that a reasonable body of medical opinion would have mentioned. Consequently, it cannot be assumed that judges will accept an argument that most doctors would not have explained a potential risk before the patient consented to undergo the procedure if, in the opinion of the judge, that risk should have been explained[1].

The General Medical Council believes that successful relationships between doctors and patients depend on trust[2]. To establish that trust, doctors must respect the autonomy of patients, including their right to decide whether or not to undergo any medical intervention even where a refusal may result in harm to themselves or in their own death. Patients must be given sufficient information, in a way that they can understand, to enable them to exercise their right to make informed decisions about their care. The Department of Health has stated that doctors are expected to be aware of the legal principles set by relevant case law in this area[3]. Doctors must take appropriate steps to find out what patients want to know and ought to know about their condition and its treatment.

Anaesthesia is a non-therapeutic intervention, with no benefit to the patient other than the benefit of allowing surgery to take place. The public perception is that it is simple and safe. The fact is that it is fairly safe (and not that simple). However, because it is perceived to be safe, is non-therapeutic and is associated from time to time with injury, allegations that inadequate information was provided by the anaesthetist have become common, particularly in relation to regional blocks.

Intensive care units (ICUs) treat the most seriously ill patients in a hospital, using techniques that may or may not have been proved to be beneficial, performing invasive interventions with significant risks of complications and using drugs that seldom have a licence for administration in the pertaining circumstances. A large proportion of the patients are unable to give consent to treatment because they are unconscious or so seriously ill that they cannot fulfil the criteria for competence. However, to date, issues of consent and information have featured only rarely in civil litigation relating to management in the ICU. For the time being at least, patients and their relatives appear to accept that ICU staff act in the best interests of patients who cannot give consent, and any litigation is directed at the standard of clinical care.

The remainder of this chapter concentrates on the principles that apply to provision of information and seeking of consent in England; the principles are the same in most other countries although detail, particularly regarding young people aged 16 and 17 years, may differ slightly (for a discussion on issues related to children and consent, see Chapter 6). Observations are included that are relevant to the practice of anaesthetists and of staff working in ICUs.

Consent in competent adults

Consent must be given voluntarily by an appropriately informed person who is competent to consent to the intervention in question.

Voluntary consent

Consent must be given voluntarily and freely, without pressure or undue influence either to accept or refuse treatment. Such pressure can come from partners or family members, or from other carers. Doctors should be alert to this possibility, and, if necessary, they should arrange to see the patient alone. The views of health-care professionals on the perceived benefits of a treatment must not lead to coercion to accept the treatment.

While competent adults have an absolute right to refuse treatment in its entirety, doctors are not obliged to treat the patient who refuses specific components of treatment if these components are important in determining the success of the treatment. Doctors have a responsibility to provide what is, in their judgement, treatment that has the most favourable predicted outcome for the patient. For example, if a patient scheduled to undergo elective oesophago-gastrectomy refused consent for insertion of a central venous catheter and arterial catheter after being told of the risks of these procedures, it would be wrong for the anaesthetist to coerce the patient into agreeing; however, if no reasonable body of opinion would support undertaking the operation without a central venous catheter and arterial catheter, then proceeding with the operation without the information that these catheters would provide would be regarded as professional misconduct. Consequently, while there must be no coercion, anaesthetists must be prepared to refuse elective treatment if the patient's decision compromises the anaesthetist's ability to provide a safe level of care. Similar arguments pertain in patients admitted to the ICU.

Provision of appropriate information

To be properly informed, a patient needs to understand in broad terms the nature and purpose of the procedure, and any relevant potential complications or side-effects. In the case of Sidaway[4], a patient who underwent surgery to the cervical spine was paralysed as a result of damage to the spinal cord. Mrs Sidaway's claim was based on the failure to warn her of the risk of damage to the cord (estimated to be a risk of less than 1%) or to warn her of a combined risk of damage to a nerve root and/or spinal cord (estimated at 2%). It was assumed that the surgeon had told her of the possibility of disturbing a nerve root, but had not mentioned the risk of spinal cord damage. It was found that a responsible body of neuro-surgeons would not have discussed death or paralysis because this would have frightened the patient. The case was eventually considered in the House of Lords, and the Law Lords, who found in favour of the hospital on a majority decision, made a number of observations.

> The doctor cannot set out to educate the patient to his own standard of medical knowledge of all the relevant factors involved. He may take the view, certainly with some patients, that the very fact of his volunteering, without being asked, information of some remote risk involved in the treatment proposed, even though he describes it as remote, may lead to that risk assuming an undue significance in the patient's calculations.

It is a matter of clinical judgement to determine what degree of disclosure of risks is best suited to assist a particular patient to make a rational choice as to whether or not to undergo a particular treatment.

> Whether or not failure to disclose a risk or cluster of risks in a particular case constitutes a breach of the doctor's duty is a matter to be decided principally on the basis of expert medical evidence. Having heard the evidence it is for the judge to decide whether a responsible body of medical opinion would have approved of non-disclosure in the circumstances of the case.

Reference to a reasonable body of medical opinion refers to what is know as the Bolam test[5] – a doctor is not guilty of negligence if his practice conformed to that of a responsible body of medical opinion held by practitioners skilled in the field in question. However, the Law Lords left it open for a judge to override expert medical opinion.

> A judge may come to the conclusion that, even in the absence of expert witnesses, disclosure of a particular risk was so obviously necessary to an informed choice on the part of the patient that no reasonably prudent medical man would fail to make it.

In December 1987, Mrs Davis underwent marsupialisation of a Bartholin's cyst. The operation was performed under general anaesthesia, but a caudal block was undertaken after she was unconscious, in order to provide intra-operative and post-operative analgesia. Post-operatively, she was unable to move her legs and had no control over her bladder. There was considerable improvement over the next 48 hours, but a neurological abnormality persisted, affecting predominantly her left foot. It was accepted that the caudal block had not been discussed with her before anaesthesia, and it was alleged that performance of the caudal block was, therefore, a trespass. The court accepted that, in 1987, a responsible body of anaesthetists would not have told a patient specifically that a caudal block would be performed after induction of general anaesthesia. Judgment was in favour of the defendants, Havering and Brentwood Health Authority. The judge rejected the suggestion made by Mrs Davis that she should have been informed of each component of her anaesthetic, saying that this sectionalised approach would encourage the 'deplorable' prospect of actions being brought in trespass rather than negligence[6]:

> If one is to treat the administration of an injection for analgesic purposes while the patient is generally anaesthetised (e.g. the caudal block) as something requiring separate consent, why should separate consent not also be sought for an injection of, for example, morphine to provide analgesia when the patient begins to come around from the general anaesthetic. . . . In my judgement, there is no realistic distinction between omitting to tell a patient that while she is under a general anaesthetic a tube will be put in her trachea and omitting to tell her that while she is under a general anaesthetic a needle will be put into her caudal region to provide post-operative analgesia.

The view of the Association of Anaesthetists of Great Britain and Ireland (AAGBI) is that patients should be informed if a local anaesthetic block is to be used[7]. *Davis v. Barking, Havering and Brentwood HA*[6] might not, therefore, help an anaesthetist sued in similar circumstances now. What is 'reasonable' to a body of medical opinion changes through time, and documents released by established bodies like the AAGBI are certainly contemporary evidence of a reasonable body of opinion.

Since *Sidaway*[4], judgments in a number of negligence cases (relating both to the provision of information and to the standard of treatment given) have shown that courts are willing to be critical of a 'responsible body' of medical opinion, particularly if that opinion does not withstand logical analysis. It is now clear that the courts will be the final arbiter of what constitutes responsible practice, particularly with regard to consent[1], although *Bolam* remains influential.

A recent Court of Appeal judgment[8] stated that it will normally be the responsibility of a doctor to inform a patient of 'a significant risk':

> If there is a significant risk which would affect the judgement of a reasonable patient, then in the normal course it is the responsibility of the doctor to inform the patient of that significant risk, if the information is needed so that

the patient can determine for him or herself as to what course he or she should adopt.

The GMC advises that doctors should do their best to find out about patients' individual needs and priorities when providing information[2]. If the patient asks specific questions about the procedure and associated risks then these should be answered truthfully. If the doctor believes that to follow these guidelines in full would have a deleterious effect on the patient's health then this view, and the reasons for it, should be recorded in the patient's notes. The mere fact that the patient might become upset by hearing the information, or might refuse treatment, is not sufficient to justify withholding the information.

The Professional Conduct Committee of the GMC paid no heed to *Bolam* when considering allegations of assault against an anaesthetist who inserted an analgesic suppository during general anaesthesia without seeking the patient's consent. The events took place in a dental surgery, and the patient was fully clothed. The Committee was told that it was not standard practice to seek specific consent for insertion of an analgesic suppository, but reached the conclusion that the patient had been assaulted[9]. Standard practice changed almost overnight.

With specific regard to anaesthesia, the AAGBI has recommended that the following factors should be considered by an anaesthetist when deciding what to explain to patients[7]:

- The gravity of the risks involved in the proposed anaesthetic technique.
- The frequency with which a complication is encountered according to the literature.
- The estimated risks of alternative techniques.
- The estimated added risks for the individual patient (e.g. as a result of concurrent disease).
- The estimated capacity of the patient to want to know, and to be able to understand, the risks.
- The degree of urgency of the proposed treatment.

It was not recommended that every risk of every component of the anaesthetic technique should be explained ('sectionalised consent'). The AAGBI believed that this would require presentation of a bewildering quantity of information, which could result in patients providing restricted consent that was entirely inappropriate. For example, a patient requiring emergency abdominal surgery might agree to general anaesthesia but not to tracheal intubation.

It was, however, recommended that anaesthetists should usually warn patients of common risks (e.g. muscle pains following administration of suxamethonium, postural headache after spinal anaesthesia), that the patient should normally be told that there is a small risk of more serious complications associated with any anaesthetic, and that the anaesthetist should provide details if asked to elaborate (e.g. regarding awareness, nerve damage, cerebral damage, death).

The AAGBI gave specific advice about the nature of information that anaesthetists should provide to patients[7]:

- The anaesthetist should explain what the patient will experience before and after anaesthesia. This includes the need to fast, administration and effects of premedication, transfer to the anaesthetic room, connection to monitors, insertion of needles and injection of anaesthetic drugs. It may be reassuring to the patient to be told that the anaesthetist will be present at all times during the operation to maintain anaesthesia and to ensure the patient's safety. Where appropriate, the need for blood transfusion should be discussed.
- Patients should be told that, post-operatively, they will awaken in a recovery room soon after the end of the operation, but they may remember nothing until they have returned to the ward. When the patient regains consciousness, there will be an oxygen mask on the face and (if appropriate) the patient will be aware that a nasogastric tube has been introduced. If appropriate, patients should be told that pain should be anticipated post-operatively. The proposed method of pain control should be explained (e.g. patient-controlled analgesia, intravenous injection of opioids in the recovery area, epidural analgesia).
- If a patient is expected to go to a high dependency unit or ICU post-operatively, then appropriate information should be given, including information relating to any invasive monitoring techniques that are planned.
- Day-stay patients in hospitals or dental surgeries must be supplied with clear and comprehensive pre- and post-operative instructions, and told that, when they leave the premises, they must be accompanied by a responsible adult.
- If a local or regional anaesthetic technique is to be used, then patients should be informed of the nature of the technique, and that numbness and/or weakness may be experienced in the first few post-operative hours. The patient should be told also that alternative techniques, including the use of general anaesthesia, may be required if the block is unsuccessful.
- If it is proposed that local or regional anaesthesia is to be used alone, then this should be explained to the patient. Some patients do not wish to remain conscious during an operation, and they may reject these techniques. In those who consent, it should be explained that they may experience some sensation during surgery, including possibly a degree of pain, even if a sedative drug is to be administered concurrently.
- If a technique of a sensitive nature, such as the insertion of an analgesic suppository, is to be employed during anaesthesia, then the patient should be informed, so that there is no anxiety afterwards if there are unusual sensations or if the residuum of a suppository is evacuated.
- Patients who are at increased risk from anaesthesia and surgery should be told the nature of the increased risk and, if possible, an estimate of the probability of the risk materialising should be provided.
- All patients should be given the opportunity to ask questions, and honest answers should be provided.
- Many questions relate to the operation. The anaesthetist should not provide information about the surgical procedure beyond his or her capability. The anaesthetist should ensure that an appropriate person discusses the procedure and answers the patient's questions before anaesthesia is induced.

Clear information is particularly important when students or trainees carry out procedures to further their own education. If the procedure will further the patient's care (e.g. inserting an intravenous cannula that will be used for administration of drugs or fluids) then, assuming the student is appropriately trained in the procedure and supervised, the fact that it is carried out by a student does not alter the nature and purpose of the procedure. It is, therefore, not a legal requirement to tell the patient that the clinician is a student, although it is good practice to do so. In contrast, where a student proposes to conduct a physical examination that is not part of the patient's care, then it is essential to explain that the purpose of the examination is to further the student's training and to seek consent for that to take place. This is particularly important if the examination is to take place during general anaesthesia.

Competence to give consent

A competent adult is a person who has reached 18 years of age, and who has the capacity to make decisions on his or her own behalf regarding treatment. That capacity is present if the patient can comprehend and retain information provided about treatment, including the consequences of having or not having the treatment; believes that information; and weighs that information in the balance to arrive at a choice[10]. No other person can consent to treatment on behalf of an adult[11]. Patients may be competent to consent to some interventions but not to others. Adults are presumed to be competent to provide consent, but, where any doubt exists, the capacity of the patient to give consent should be assessed[12]. This assessment and the conclusions drawn from it should be recorded in the patient's notes.

A patient's capacity to comprehend and believe information, and to make a balanced choice, may be affected by factors such as confusion, panic, shock, fatigue, pain or medication. However, the existence of such factors should not be assumed automatically to render the patient incapable of providing consent. An apparently unreasonable decision by the patient does not necessarily imply that the patient lacks competence. The competent patient is entitled to make a decision that is based on their own belief or value system, even if it is perceived by others to be irrational, as long as the patient understands the consequences of that decision.

Additional procedures

During an operation it may become evident that the patient would benefit from an additional procedure that was not within the scope of the original consent. If it would be unreasonable to delay the procedure until the patient regains consciousness, it may be justified to perform the procedure on the grounds that it is in the patient's best interests. For example, this could apply to insertion of invasive monitoring catheters in a patient who bled unexpectedly, or insertion of an epidural catheter for post-operative pain control if the nature of the operation changed. However, the procedure should not be performed merely because it is convenient. In addition, if a patient has refused specific procedures before anaesthesia, then this refusal must be respected. The use of additional procedures without consent might have to be defended. It is no defence to have a signed consent form that specifies 'and anything else deemed necessary at the time'. Rather it will be necessary to show that the additional procedures could not reasonably have been foreseen and that urgent measures were necessary to protect the life or health of the patient.

Consent to video recordings and clinical photography

Photographs and video recordings of treatment may be used both as a medical record and as a tool for teaching, audit or research. The Department of Health does not regard it as necessary to obtain consent for images that will be used solely as part of the medical record. However, if the images are to be used for teaching, audit, research or publication, patients must be made aware that they can refuse without their care being compromised. It is now standard practice to obtain written consent for images to be taken for any purpose other than to form part of the medical record.

Who can obtain consent?

The clinician who provides treatment has a duty to ensure that the patient has given valid consent. The task of seeking consent may be delegated to another health-care professional provided that the individual is suitably trained and qualified. The individual who seeks consent must have sufficient knowledge of the proposed treatment and its associated risks and complications because of the need to provide appropriate information and to answer questions accurately. It is likely that competency-based training of doctors will include tests of competency to obtain consent for specific procedures as well as competency in performing the procedure, and that only those who have proved their competence at obtaining consent will be authorised to have that responsibility delegated to them. There will be situations in which other health-care professionals, usually nurses, may, with appropriate training, be deemed competent to obtain consent for surgical or anaesthetic procedures.

When should consent be sought?

The seeking and giving of consent is usually a process, rather than a one-off event. For major surgical interventions, it is good practice where possible to seek the patient's consent to the proposed procedure well in advance, when there is time to respond to the patient's questions and provide adequate information. The Department of Health has recently introduced new consent forms for use in hospitals in England and Wales[2]. The intention is that consent for elective surgery will be obtained at the outpatient clinic when the patient is put on the waiting list for operation. In addition to the explanation and information provided by the surgeon, printed leaflets containing detailed information about the proposed procedure, and about the anaesthetic techniques that will most probably be employed (general anaesthesia, spinal/epidural anaesthesia, local anaesthesia), will be given to the patient. The patient will be given a copy of the consent form. On the back of the form is further information advising patients that they may ask specific questions, such as the experience of the surgeon in undertaking the operation, and the incidences of complications in his or her practice. When the patient is admitted for surgery, he or she must sign a separate section of the consent form, acknowledging that no further information is required, and confirming that consent has been given. Clinicians should then check, before the procedure starts, that the patient still consents.

Although some surgical patients are seen by an anaesthetist at a pre-operative assessment clinic, the large majority first meet an anaesthetist less than 24 hours before anaesthesia and surgery, and, with current admission practices, not uncommonly in the anaesthetic room immediately before the procedure. The Department of Health regards it as unacceptable in elective procedures for the patient to receive no information about anaesthesia until the pre-operative visit from the anaesthetist, on the grounds that, at such a late stage, the patient will not be in a position to make an informed decision about whether or not to undergo anaesthesia[3].

Patients should therefore either receive a general leaflet about anaesthesia in out-patients, or have the opportunity to discuss anaesthesia in a pre-assessment clinic. The anaesthetist should ensure that the discussion with the patient and their consent is documented in the anaesthetic record, in the patient's notes or on the consent form.

If general anaesthesia or sedation is required for dental treatment, the General Dental Council holds the dentist responsible for ensuring that the patient (or, in the case of children, a parent) has all the necessary information about the benefits and risks of anaesthesia at the time that the decision is taken to recommend the treatment[12]. If an anaesthetist is involved at the time of treatment, then it is his or her responsibility to ensure that the risks and benefits are understood by the patient, and to obtain consent for anaesthesia.

Form of consent

Consent may be given verbally or non-verbally: an example of non-verbal consent would be where a patient, after receiving appropriate information, holds out an arm for their blood pressure to be taken. Verbal consent is the norm in respect of anaesthesia. The AAGBI did not believe that there was any virtue in requiring the patient to sign a consent form for anaesthesia, or a separate section on the surgical consent form relating specifically to anaesthesia, provided that the anaesthetist made a record of the anaesthetic techniques (e.g. general anaesthesia, regional anaesthesia, local anaesthesia or a combination) that had been discussed with and agreed by the patient, and listed the material risks that had been explained[7]. There is a danger that, if written consent is required for any procedure, then health-care professionals concentrate their attention on obtaining a signature on a form rather than ensuring that the principles of consent (agreement to treatment after consideration of all information that the patient considers to be relevant) have been achieved.

The Department of Health has recently produced templates for consent forms for hospital patients[3]. There are three versions of the standard consent form: Form 1 for adults or competent children; Form 2 for parental consent for a child or young person; and Form 3 when the patient will remain alert throughout the procedure. Form 4 is applicable to an adult patient who does not have the capacity to give or withhold consent.

Research and innovative treatment

Clinical research can be conducted only if the study has been approved by a properly constituted Research Ethics Committee (REC). Before approving a study, the REC will take into account the validity of the research, and the welfare and dignity of the patient[13]. Ethics committee approval does not, however, absolve the clinicians carrying out the research from ethical or legal responsibility for their own actions.

Consent is normally required before a patient can be included in a research study. Sufficient information must be given regarding the nature of the research, its purpose, the possible hazards and benefits (if any) and the degree of risk involved in participation. The information should be presented in a manner, form and at such a time as to permit the patient to consider as fully as possible all the relevant issues and to reach an informed decision about whether to participate or not. Consent must be voluntary, and it should not be influenced by a desire to avoid the disapproval of the researcher or by any form of inducement. It must be made clear to patients that there is no obligation to participate, and that they may withdraw from the study at any time without affecting the standard of clinical care provided.

If the treatment being offered is of an experimental nature, but not part of a formal research trial, this fact must be clearly explained to patients before their consent is sought, along with information about standard alternatives. The patient should be told about existing evidence about the effectiveness and possible side-effects or hazards of the treatment, based not only on the practitioner's own experience but also on experience and reports from other centres.

New unlicensed drugs that are undergoing clinical trials are normally administered only as part of a formal research investigation, and the guidelines above should be followed. Indemnity from the manufacturer should be obtained in relation to adverse events occurring as a consequence of administration of the drug. This indemnity does not cover negligence on the part of the prescriber or the person who administers the drug. All drug trials that involve unlicensed drugs, or drugs used outside the terms of the Product Licence, require permission from the Medicines Control Agency.

Duration of consent

In general, consent remains valid for an indefinite duration unless it is withdrawn by the patient. However, the GMC recommends that a doctor should inform the patient if new information has become available about the proposed intervention after consent was sought but before the intervention is undertaken, and that consent is reconfirmed[2]. If the patient's condition has changed significantly in the intervening time, it may be necessary to seek consent again, on the basis that the likely benefits or risks of the intervention may also have changed.

Refusal of consent

Competent adult patients have a right to refuse treatment with or without good reason. If a competent adult makes a voluntary and informed decision to refuse treatment this decision **must** be respected, except in circumstances defined by the *Mental Health Act (1983)*. This is the case even where refusal of consent may result in the death of the patient[14] or the death of an unborn child, whatever the stage of the pregnancy[15].

If a patient refuses to consent to the anaesthetic technique that the anaesthetist believes to be the most appropriate, or refuses a form of treatment in the ICU that the staff believe to be the most appropriate, then reasonable attempts can be made to persuade the patient that the proposed technique or procedure carries the least risk of adverse sequelae. The advantages and disadvantages of the proposed procedure in relation to alternatives, and the reasons for the advice, should be explained clearly. However, it is not acceptable to coerce patients into accepting a specific form of treatment.

Occasionally, a refusal of treatment appears so bizarre or irrational that it raises the possibility of mental disorder. If this is considered to be a possibility, then a psychiatric opinion should be sought.

Withdrawal of consent

A competent patient is entitled to withdraw consent at any time, including during the performance of a procedure. In anaesthetic practice, this may occur immediately before induction of anaesthesia, during the performance of a local or regional block, or during operations performed under local or regional anaesthesia. If a patient does object during treatment, the procedure should be stopped, if this is possible. The reasons for the patient's concerns should be established, and the consequences of not completing the procedure explained. If stopping the procedure would put the life of the patient at risk, it is probably best to continue until this risk no longer applies.

Assessing capacity to give or withdraw consent during a procedure may be difficult because pain, panic and shock may diminish the capacity to consent. In anaesthetic practice, this arises most commonly in the obstetric unit (see Chapter 10). If capacity is lacking, it may sometimes be justified to continue in the patient's best interests, although this should not be used as an excuse to ignore distress.

Advance statements or directives

Some patients elect to express their wishes about future treatment in the event that they may subsequently become incompetent to provide consent or to express their wishes. The most common example relating to anaesthetic practice is a directive indicating refusal to undergo surgery for advanced and irreversible malignant disease, or an intercurrent surgical condition in the presence of a severely incapacitating and progressive degenerative disease. Many Jehovah's Witnesses carry with them an advance statement forbidding the administration of blood or blood components[16]. Patients may have indicated in an advance statement that they do not wish heroic efforts at resuscitation to be made in the event of a life-threatening illness, particularly if the long-term prognosis is poor even if resuscitation is successful, and these wishes must be considered if admission to an ICU is contemplated.

An advance statement is legally binding upon doctors when it expresses refusal of treatment in circumstances that the patient had anticipated. When a situation falls fully within the terms of the advance statement, then clinicians should respect its terms unless there is evidence that the patient may have changed his or her mind since signing it.

An advance statement cannot authorise doctors to do anything outside the law, or compel them to carry out a specific form of treatment. In particular, an advance statement cannot permit a clinician to commit an act intended to end a patient's life.

If there is doubt about the validity of an advance statement, a Court ruling should be sought. A health-care professional must not override a valid and applicable advance statement on the grounds of a personal conscientious objection to the terms of the statement.

It has been suggested that as a matter of public policy individuals should not be able to refuse in advance measures that are essential to keep a patient comfortable[17]. This 'basic' or 'essential' care includes keeping the patient warm, clean and free from distressing symptoms such as breathlessness, vomiting and severe pain. However, some patients may prefer to tolerate some discomfort if this means they remain more alert and able to respond to family and friends.

Force-feeding a patient or the use of artificial nutrition and hydration does not form part of 'basic' or 'essential' care. A competent individual has the right to choose to refuse food or hydration. Towards the end of such a period of starvation, a patient is likely to lose capacity. The courts have ruled that if, when competent to do so, an individual has indicated clearly a wish to refuse food or water until death occurs, then the person cannot be force-fed or fed artificially when incompetent.*

Self-harm

Patients who have deliberately harmed themselves present special difficulties to health-care professionals if they refuse treatment. If the patient is able to communicate, an assessment of mental capacity should be made as soon as possible. A patient who is judged not to be competent may be treated on the basis of

---

*If the patient is refusing food as a result of mental disorder and is detained under the Mental Health Act (1983), different considerations may apply.

temporary incapacity (see below). Patients who have attempted suicide and are unconscious should be given emergency treatment if any doubt exists about either their intentions or their capacity when they took the decision to attempt suicide.

However, competent patients have the right to refuse treatment. The Department of Health recommends that a psychiatric assessment should be obtained if a competent patient who has harmed him/herself refuses treatment. If the use of the *Mental Health Act (1983)* is not appropriate, then the refusal must be respected. If practitioners have good reason to believe that a patient genuinely intended to end his or her life and was competent when that decision was taken, and are satisfied that the *Mental Health Act (1983)* is not applicable, then treatment should not be forced on the patient although attempts should be made to encourage him or her to accept help.

Adults without capacity

Under English law, no other person can consent to treatment on behalf of any adult, including adults who are unable to give consent for themselves ('incapable' adults)[11]. There are, however, circumstances in which treatment can be given to incapable adults. The key principle concerning treatment of the incapable adult is that of the person's best interests.

The courts have identified certain circumstances when referral should be made to them for a ruling on lawfulness before a procedure is undertaken. Circumstances relevant to anaesthesia and intensive care are sterilisation for contraceptive purposes and withdrawal of nutrition and hydration from a patient in a persistent vegetative state.

In *Re F*[11], the House of Lords considered the power of a court to authorise sterilisation of an adult woman who did not have the capacity to give consent; she was 36 years old but had the mental capacity of a child of 4 years. She had become involved in a relationship but medical staff felt that a pregnancy would be 'disastrous from a psychiatric point of view'. The House of Lords concluded that, in these circumstances, sterilisation was permissible and lawful because it was in the patient's 'best interests'. 'Best interests' was to be taken in a wide sense so as to include public interest, but in the area of non-therapeutic sterilisation, was not to include the convenience of those responsible for the patient's care.

> The overriding consideration is that [doctors] should act in the best interests of the person who suffers from the misfortune of being prevented by incapacity from deciding for himself what should be done to his own body, in his own best interests.

Females who become pregnant incur risks associated with pregnancy and delivery, and these risks are avoided if sterilisation is performed; this is not so in the case of males. An application was made by the mother of a young male adult with Down's syndrome to authorise his sterilisation because there was a possibility that he might have sexual intercourse and cause a pregnancy[18]. It was unlikely that he would be able to tolerate vasectomy under local anaesthesia and, therefore, he would be subjected to the finite, although very small, risks associated with general anaesthesia. The Court decided that it was not in the patient's best interests to be sterilised, and public interest or the interest of females whom he might impregnate was irrelevant, so the application was rejected.

The doctrine of 'best interests' was examined again by the House of Lords in the case of a victim of the Hillsborough Disaster who was in a persistent vegetative state as a result of the injuries that he had sustained[19]. The House of Lords held that:

- The object of medical treatment and care was to benefit the patient. A large body of responsible medical opinion considered that the continuation of a persistent vegetative state was not for the benefit of the patient. The principle of the sanctity of life was not violated by ceasing to give medical treatment to which the patient had not consented and which conferred no benefit upon him.
- The doctors responsible for the patient were neither under a duty, nor entitled, to continue the medical care because the patient had no further interest in being kept alive.

It was concluded that treatment could be withdrawn. The Law Lords indicated, however, that until a body of experience and practice had been built up, it was desirable that applications should be made to the Court when medical staff considered that continued treatment of a patient in a persistent vegetative state no longer conferred a benefit upon him.

Although many forms of treatment can be undertaken on individuals who are not competent to provide consent without referral to the Court, the treatment must be appropriate. Medical staff undertaking the procedure must ensure that the treatment is in a patient's 'best interest', and is not being undertaken primarily for the advantage of relatives or carers. Action in the patient's best interest is also subject to the *Bolam* standard.

Temporary incapacity

An adult who usually has capacity may become temporarily incapable, for example, whilst under a general anaesthetic or sedation, or as a result of confusion, panic, shock, fatigue, pain or medication after a road traffic accident. Unless a valid advance refusal of treatment is applicable to the circumstances, the law permits interventions to be made that are necessary and no more than is reasonably required in the patient's best interests pending the recovery of capacity. If a medical intervention is thought to be in the patient's best interests but can be delayed until the patient recovers capacity and can consent to (or refuse) the intervention, it must be delayed until that time.

Permanent or long-standing incapacity

If an adult has long-standing or permanent incapacity, it is lawful to undertake any procedure that is in the person's 'best interests'. Treatment in the patient's best interests is not confined to life-preserving procedures but includes those that will improve health or well-being, as well as much wider welfare considerations. A standard consent form should not be signed by the relatives or doctor. It is good practice to note in the medical records or on the new Consent Form 4[3] why the treatment was believed to be in the patient's best interests. It is also advisable to discuss the proposed treatment with relatives. Relatives of patients who were previously competent may be able to indicate what the patient's probable wishes would have been. If the agreement of the relatives of any incompetent patient is sought and obtained then it is less likely that any legal challenge to the validity of a decision to carry out the procedure or treatment will occur.

Fluctuating capacity

In some patients, capacity fluctuates. In such cases, it should be possible during periods of capacity to establish the patient's views about any clinical intervention that may be necessary during a period of incapacity and to record these views. If the patient does not make any relevant advance refusal, treatment during periods of incapacity should accord with the principles for treating the temporarily incapacitated (see above).

Research

This is an extremely difficult area, which creates problems when attempting to undertake research in the ICU (among other places). There is no case law in England, and this is, therefore, as much a question of ethics as law.

The strict legal position is that only a court can authorise medical treatment on an adult who is incompetent to provide consent, unless the treatment is in the patient's 'best interests'. The purpose of undertaking clinical research is usually to establish whether a new form of treatment is beneficial, or to compare two forms of treatment. The new treatment may be beneficial, but it may not. In a randomised comparative study, the patient may or may not be given the new treatment. Consequently, in the large majority of clinical trials, participation cannot be in the patient's 'best interests'.

However, some advances in medical treatment may be beneficial to groups of patients comprising predominantly those who are not competent to give consent (e.g. children and patients in an ICU). If clinical trials cannot be undertaken, then large numbers of these patients, in the future, may be deprived of a form of treatment that may reduce morbidity or mortality.

Many forms of treatment in the ICU have developed with little evidence base, and it may be predicted before a clinical trial, for example, on the basis of pilot studies, that those patients who receive the new treatment are likely to benefit. It may, therefore, be argued that there is a possibility that taking part in the trial will be in the patient's 'best interests', and that participation will not be against the patient's interests because the alternative to the new treatment will be a standard treatment.

It has been suggested that it can be ethical to perform research which involves minimal intervention on incapable adults, if certain stringent conditions are met:

the research must be approved by the relevant Research Ethics Committee; it must relate to the condition from which the incapable adult is suffering; and it must be demonstrated that the research is not against the patient's interests[20,21]. Some research in ICUs may involve more than minimal intervention; ethically, it may be appropriate to undertake such research subject to these conditions and provided that the research could not be conducted instead on patients capable of giving consent. Many Research Ethics Committees insist that patients who have been recruited to a research project while incapable of giving consent, and who subsequently recover competence to provide consent, are informed of their participation in the research project. In addition, many Research Ethics Committees insist that participation of a patient incapable of providing consent is conducted with the assent of the relatives; this minimises the risk of subsequent legal action.

The position concerning research that does not have the *potential* immediately to benefit the person's health is a legally uncharted area. This type of research should never be undertaken on incapable patients if it is possible instead to carry out the research on persons capable of giving consent.

Mental Health Act (1983)

Treatment for mental disorder may proceed without obtaining the patient's consent if the patient is liable to be detained under the *Mental Health Act (1983)*. This Act does not contain provisions to enable treatment of physical disorders without consent, either for detained patients, or for people who may be suffering from mental disorder but who are not detained under the Mental Health Act, unless the physical disorder arises from the mental disorder, or is judged to be contributing to the mental disorder.

Neither the existence of a mental disorder nor the fact of detention under the Mental Health Act should give rise to an assumption of incapacity. The patient's capacity must be assessed in every case in relation to the particular decision being made. The capacity of a person with a mental disorder may fluctuate.

Conclusions

Consent must be sought from most patients for anaesthesia. It is the duty of doctors to give the patient appropriately full information, but there is no obligation to explain every detail of what is proposed. The extent of detail provided is a matter for the clinical judgement of the doctor, bearing in mind any relevant advice from professional bodies. In the event of a dispute, each case will be considered on the basis of the individual facts.

In the ICU, most procedures are undertaken on patients who are unable to consent, either through the effects of their illness or the administration of potent drugs. Staff must consider the best interests of the patient at all times, and particularly when an invasive procedure is being contemplated. Good communication with relatives is crucial in minimising the risk of subsequent complaints.

References

1. *Bolitho* v. *Hackney HA* [1993] 4 Med. LR 381
2. General Medical Council. Seeking patients' consent: the ethical considerations. London: GMC, 1999
3. Department of Health. Good practice in consent implementation guide: consent to examination or treatment. London: DOH, 2001
4. *Sidaway* v. *Board of Governors of Bethlem Royal Hospital and the Maudsley Hospital* [1985] AC 871
5. *Bolam* v. *Friern Hospital Management Committee* [1957] 1 WLR 582
6. *Davis* v. *Barking, Havering and Brentwood HA* [1994] 4 Med LR 85
7. Association of Anaesthetists of Great Britain and Ireland. Information and Consent for Anaesthesia. London: AAGBI, 1999
8. *Pearce* v. *United Bristol Healthcare NHS Trust* [1999] 48 BMLR 118
9. Mitchell J. A fundamental problem of consent. Br Med J 1995; 310: 43–8
10. *Re: C (Refusal of Medical Treatment) [1994] 1 FLR 31*
11. *Re F* [1989] 2 WLR 1025; [1989] 2 All ER 545
12. General Dental Council. Maintaining Standards: Guidance to Dentists on Professional and Personal Conduct. London: General Dental Council, Revision November 1998.
13. Department of Health. Briefing Pack for Research Ethics Committee Members. London: DOH, 1997
14. *Ms B* v. *An NHS Hospital Trust* [2002] EWHC 429 9fam
15. *Re MB (Medical Treatment)* [1997] 2 FLR 426
16. Association of Anaesthetists of Great Britain and Ireland. Management of Anaesthesia for Jehovah's Witnesses. London: AAGBI, 1999
17. British Medical Association. Advance statements about medical treatment. London: BMA Publishing Group, 1995
18. *Re A* (Male Sterilisation) [2000] 1 FLR 549, 557
19. *Airedale NHS Trust* v. *Bland* [1993] 1 All ER 821 (HL)
20. Medical Research Council. The ethical conduct of research on the mentally incapacitated. London: MRC, 1991
21. The Royal College of Physicians of London. Guidelines on the practice of ethics committees in medical research involving human subjects. 3rd edn. London: Royal College of Physicians, 1996

Fitness to Practise, Self-Regulation and Clinical Governance in Anaesthesia   **3**

David Hatch

Introduction and history

Doctors have always recognised the importance of keeping up-to-date and ensuring fitness to practise, and a commitment to this professional obligation was implicit within the Hippocratic oath in the fifth century BC. The main purpose of the establishment of the early professional societies, and later the foundation of the first of the Royal Colleges, was the acknowledged need to set professional standards and to ensure their maintenance by a system of self-regulation. The Society of Apothecaries became the first professional body in the UK to establish an organised system of education, qualification and registration when its Charter of Medical Reform received the Royal Assent in 1815.

It was not long after the introduction of anaesthesia that John Snow recognised the importance of establishing professional standards of practice for this young speciality, lighting a torch that was carried on by Hewitt and others until the present day. Hewitt, a founder member of the Society of Anaesthetists in 1893, recognised the need for disciplinary powers to support professional self-regulation and asked the General Medical Council (GMC) in 1901 to consider the desirability of including anaesthetics in the medical curriculum. He also attempted unsuccessfully to achieve legislation restricting the administration of anaesthetics to doctors. The failure of this attempt was largely brought about by the strong dental lobby, which was not overcome until 1998. Other professionally led initiatives designed to improve the practice of anaesthesia include the establishment of an anaesthetic section of the Royal Society of Medicine, the founding of the Association of Anaesthetists of Great Britain and Ireland primarily for the purpose of introducing a diploma of anaesthetics, the founding of anaesthetic journals and the establishment of the Faculty of Anaesthetists of the Royal College of Surgeons of England (now the Royal College of Anaesthetists).

Despite continuing initiatives by professional anaesthetic bodies and the commitment of most individual anaesthetists to the maintenance of high standards of practice, more needs to be done. Recent high profile examples of doctors whose professional standards have been seriously deficient have been given extensive coverage by the news media. The fact that these doctors have, in some cases, been allowed to practise for several years despite their serious deficiencies being known to close colleagues has been a source of justifiable concern, both to the government and the public. Although the most recent surveys suggest that public confidence in doctors remains high, the ability of the profession to regulate itself in a way that protects patients from dangerous members of the profession has been increasingly questioned. The public scrutiny that has occurred in recent years has highlighted the weaknesses and limitations of the professional initiatives summarised above. The Royal Colleges have developed excellent training programmes leading to speciality recognition within each field, but they have devoted far less time to life-long learning, continuing education and professional development. The limitations of voluntary, unstructured continuing medical education – undertaken by the committed majority and avoided by those who may be in most need of it – are gradually being addressed. The need to provide evidence that continuing professional development programmes have a significant effect on clinical practice is now also widely recognised, and anaesthesia is the first specialty to begin to define core topics in which individuals need to demonstrate that they are keeping up to date.

Professionally led regulation

The need for medical practice to be supported by a regulatory body with statutory disciplinary powers was recognised in the establishment of the GMC in 1858. However, until as recently as 1980 the GMC disciplinary committee was limited to the consideration of allegations of 'infamous conduct', now known as 'serious professional misconduct'. Virtually all the cases heard by this committee related to allegations of criminal behaviour by doctors or serious abuse of the doctor/patient relationship, and the GMC played virtually no role in relation to doctors whose professional clinical standards of care were unsatisfactory, unless they amounted to criminal negligence. In 1980, following the successful Sick Doctor Scheme introduced by the Association of Anaesthetists of Great Britain and Ireland, the GMC introduced its Health Procedures designed to deal with doctors whose performance was seriously affected by their own state of health. These procedures deal largely with psychosis and drug or alcohol abuse in doctors who either have no insight into their health problems or are not prepared to admit to them. Designed primarily to protect the public, these procedures also allow the possibility of the doctor receiving remedial treatment and rehabilitation.

For some years, the GMC has been aware of the inability of its Professional Conduct Committee (PCC) to deal with doctors whose patterns of clinical performance are seriously deficient, since this committee deals only with specific allegations. If these allegations are not proved, no further action can be taken against the doctor even if, in the course of the hearing, other facts emerge that give seirous concern about clinical performance. For example, if an allegation that an anaesthetist failed to conduct an essential pre-operative evaluation of a patient is not proved at the PCC, no further action can be taken even if it has become apparent during the hearing that the doctor keeps no records. For this and other reasons, the GMC obtained the legislation required to introduce its performance procedures from 1 July 1997. Under these procedures doctors whose clinical performance is alleged to be seriously deficient may be required to undergo a comprehensive global assessment of their clinical practice. This assessment, carried out where possible at the doctor's place of work, is conducted by two medical assessors from the same area of clinical practice as the doctor being assessed and one non-medical assessor, all appointed and trained by the GMC. The assessment, which is tailored to the doctor's actual practice, examines all areas of the doctor's practice by a structured assessment of record keeping, the use of case-based interviews with the doctor using a selected sub-set of case notes, third party interviews with anyone who can shed light on the doctor's performance and an assessment of the environmental constraints that may affect the doctor's practice. The GMC recognises that performance embraces attitudes as well as knowledge and skills[1]. However, where doubts arise about the adequacy of a doctor's knowledge or skills a separate assessment of clinical competence is carried out using standardised methods of testing. The performance procedures are again designed primarily to protect the public, with the GMC having the powers to restrict or suspend a doctor's registration. They also provide an opportunity for retraining of doctors where this is possible. At present the opportunities for retraining are extremely limited, and some of the ethical issues related to retraining, such as how to obtain fully informed consent from patients, are proving difficult to resolve. It is to be hoped that the Government's recently established National Clinical Assessment Agency, to which doctors may be referred before their deficiencies become serious, will be able to provide more opportunities and resources for retraining than are currently available.

One of the GMC's most important recent initiatives has been the publication of its booklet *Good Medical Practice* (*GMP*)[2]. This, for the first time, gives clear guidance to doctors about the standards required of them by the profession. The guidance covers not only clinical practice but also the professional obligation upon doctors to keep up-to-date and to take appropriate action when they suspect that their own or a colleague's performance may be a source of danger to patients. The GMC has also issued guidance to managers and others on how to apply the principles in *GMP*. The booklet also sets standards for relationships with patients and colleagues, for teaching and training, probity and health. Some doctors have been under the misapprehension that *GMP* is a statement of the ideals to which doctors should aspire rather than a guide to the basic principles of competence, care and conduct expected of all doctors by the profession. The third edition (2001) of *GMP*[2] makes it clear that serious or persistent failures to meet the standards in the booklet may put a doctor's registration at risk.

In 1997, the Royal College of Anaesthetists and the Association of Anaesthetists of Great Britain and Ireland set up a joint working party to respond to the then Chief Medical Officer's request for all acute clinical services to produce benchmarks of good practice for their specialty. The working party produced *Good Practice: a Guide for Departments of Anaesthesia*[3], the first of a series of specialty-specific interpretations of *GMP* produced by the medical royal colleges and specialist associations. In their own document the Royal College of General Practitioners has attempted to list the attributes of both an excellent GP and an unacceptable one.

Good Medical Practice is one of a number of initiatives taken by the GMC in recent years. The decision to increase the non-medical membership of the Council from 10% to 25% in 1996 and the introduction of the Specialist Register in 1997 are two other examples.

Clinical governance

Clinical governance, has been defined as a 'framework through which National Health Service (NHS) organisations are accountable for continuously improving the quality of their services and safeguarding high standards of care by creating an environment in which excellence in clinical care will flourish'[4]. Through it, the current UK government aims to assure and improve the quality and safety of clinical services. It sets out a three-pronged approach to quality improvement comprising:

- Clear national quality standards set by a new National Institute for Clinical Excellence (NICE) promoting clinical excellence and cost-effectiveness through guidance and audit and developing a programme of evidence-based National Service Frameworks (NSFs), which set out what patients can expect to receive in major care areas or disease groups. NSFs have, so far, been developed for cancer services and children's intensive care. Others are being developed for diabetes, mental health, services for older people and coronary heart disease.
- Dependable local delivery through systems of clinical governance in local organisations, including mandatory audit.
- Strong monitoring mechanisms: a new statutory Commission for Health Improvement to monitor local systems, offer support where necessary and investigate persistent problems. A Performance Assessment Framework will publish comparative results from different units over a wide range of conditions, and there will be a national survey of NHS patient and user experience.

Government expects that serious failures will become uncommon, similar kinds of failure will not recur, incidents in one part of the country will not be repeated elsewhere, systems will be in place to minimise the risk of serious failures happening and less serious incidents will be reported and monitored by a new mandatory national adverse event reporting scheme. Current evidence in relation to errors (such as inadvertent intrathecal administration of vincristine sulphate or incompatible blood transfusion) suggests that much work needs to be done if these expectations are to be realised.

The concepts of professional self-regulation and life-long learning are both embedded in the Clinical Governance Quality Framework. The Government is addressing the performance of individuals by introducing a system of compulsory annual appraisal, regular review of performance and personal development plans for all doctors working in the NHS. In England and Wales, where there are doubts or concerns about clinical performance that cannot be resolved locally, the employer will be able to refer the doctor to the newly established National Clinical Assessment Authority. If there is a clear and immediate risk to patients, the doctor may be referred to the GMC. Other indications for referral to the GMC include cases where local action has failed or is impractical, or has wider implications.

It is essential that managerially led and professionally led initiatives fit together like pieces of a jigsaw. The Chief Medical Officer is on record as saying we are not playing 'one club golf', and no individual initiative will provide the improved quality of health care that the public now expects. Indeed, many now feel that the public have unrealistic expectations of the health care services that can be provided, and that these expectations have been fuelled both by Government and the media. It is certainly difficult for many people to understand that there will always be a spectrum of performance both by individuals and by groups so that, assuming a normally distributed population, 50% of doctors will always be below average! Even if the whole population improves its standards there will be a natural tendency for patients to wish to be treated by the best doctors and for the worst to be disciplined or even removed from practice (Fig. 3.1). The introduction of league tables does nothing to counter this misconception and, indeed, may enhance it as has been seen in the teaching profession. What then, one may ask, can be done to resolve this dilemma? It seems to me that the solution must lie in the identification of absolute, criterion-referenced standards wherever possible and in finding a way of enabling the public to help set these standards and, thus, identify with them. For this reason it would appear that non-medical involvement in standard setting is an essential priority for the future.

Some Royal Colleges, including the Royal College of Anaesthetists, have established patient liaison groups: a laudable development. However, in many cases, they

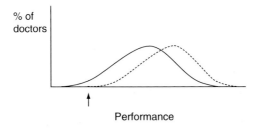

Figure 3.1. The performance distribution curve. Even if the performance of the whole population improves, some doctors will perform better than others. It is essential to identify criterion-referenced minimum standards (arrowed) acceptable to the profession and the public.

are small and not fully involved in decision making. There are also difficult issues concerning the selection and training of lay people, which are only just beginning to be addressed. With the increasing non-medical participation explicitly required by the GMC and the Government, these issues are becoming increasingly urgent. Though some health-care professionals may feel threatened by the increased involvement of lay people in decision making those who have experienced this involvement rapidly come to appreciate its value. A past chairman of the Royal College of Anaesthetists' Patient Liaison Group, Charlotte Williamson, has pointed out that:

> . . . the patient representatives' task of representation is not different from that of, say, an anaesthetist representing anaesthetic interests and values to a group of obstetricians: each has different knowledge bases, priorities and perspectives that can be drawn upon and, if necessary, explained. Compared with health professionals, patient representatives' knowledge base is less well defined, more eclectic and more dependent on the resources and experience available to the individual representative.[5]

Errors in medicine

The major advances in medicine that have occurred in recent years have not only given doctors the power to confer great benefits on patients, but also the ability to cause great harm. In this context, human errors may have much more serious implications for our patients. There have been relatively few studies of the incidence of error in health-care, and most data come from the United States[6] and Australia[7]. The latest UK analyses suggest that an estimated 850 000 adverse events might occur each year in the NHS hospital sector, resulting in a £2 billion direct cost in additional hospital days alone. Around half of these adverse events are thought to be avoidable. Experience from the serious incident reporting system run by one of the NHS Executive's Regional Offices suggests that, nationally, at least 2500 adverse events occur a year that are potentially serious enough to register on such systems. There is almost certainly a significant under-reporting of such events.

In defining the incidence of errors, it is important to understand what we mean by a medical error. In developing the GMC's performance procedures, it became clear that there was a well-recognised error rate in reporting of X-rays and histopathological material, even in the best practices. Whilst the cost of reducing this error rate to zero would be prohibitively high, it should surely be a consideration when determining whether an individual doctor has been performing at a seriously deficient level. Equally, not all errors are regarded as equally serious, even though they may cause harm to patients. For example, if a surgeon fails to diagnose acute appendicitis in the presence of a clear medical history and physical signs, this would be regarded as a serious mistake. If, on the other hand, a surgeon removes a normal appendix unnecessarily, this is regarded as unremarkable, even though the patient has suffered an unnecessary operation.

The largest number of adverse events in the published data are drug related, followed by wound infection and technical complications. Many of these, however, are unpredictable and impossible to prevent, such as allergic reactions to drugs to which the patient had no previous known exposure. Some are complications that might have been avoidable, and others result from errors in administration or monitoring. The percentage of adverse events due to negligence is highest in relation to diagnostic or therapeutic mishaps. Only a small percentage of adverse events that harm patients are due to the serious deficiencies in individual doctors that would bring them before the GMC.

Given the complex nature of medical practice and the multiplicity of interventions that each patient receives, a high error rate is perhaps not surprising. Patients in intensive care may receive around 200 interventions of one sort or another each day, so that an average of 1.7 errors per patient per day, as reported in one publication[8], must be seen in the context of staff functioning at a 99% level of proficiency. However, the 1% failure rate is substantially higher than would be tolerated in other hazardous fields of activity, such as aviation.

In a well-managed system, there should be several layers of defence separating the hazards from the losses. James Reason, one of the UK's leading researchers in the field of systems failures and error, has studied a number of major non-medical disasters such as the Challenger space-flight, the Zeebrugge cross-channel ferry disaster and the fire at King's Cross underground station in London[9]. In each case he identified what he called active errors by individuals: the unsafe acts committed by those at the sharp end whose effects are felt most immediately. They tend to occupy the spotlight in any investigation. He also, however, identified in every case latent errors, whose adverse consequences may lie dormant within the system for a long time. He likens these to resident pathogens within the human body that only become evident when they combine with other factors to breach the system's defences. They may include fatigue, staff shortages, lack of experience or inadequate equipment. They are often more difficult to identify and less satisfactory to deal with, since usually no individual can be held accountable. In reality, therefore, there are always holes in the defence layers: some caused by active failures of individuals and others by latent conditions. Serious danger only arises when a set of holes opens up in the defences, allowing a brief window of accident opportunity. The more protective layers there are, the safer the system.

It may be helpful to learn from the airline industry's approach to error management. Interestingly, although the error rate in medicine is clearly high, it may not be significantly different from that in aviation[10]. The reason that errors in aviation virtually never lead to disaster appears to be that each event is promptly recognised and corrected, and, over the years, many layers of defences have been built into the system. All near miss mid-air collisions, which are reported to occur more than 5000 times a year, are automatically logged and investigated. Pilots must undertake performance-testing examinations in a simulator on a regular basis. In short, the airline industry is a good example of an industry whose basic approach is the acknowledgement that even good individuals will sometimes make mistakes, and which takes steps to deal with them in a blame-free way. Such checks and balances as are required to minimise the chance of mistakes leading to adverse outcomes are built into the risk management systems. A system-based approach in anaesthesia has reduced the mortality in anaesthesia from 1:10 000 to 1:200 000 in recent years[11]. The increasing use of patient simulators may reduce it further. In medicine generally, however, the basic approach continues to be to rely on individuals not to make mistakes, or to try to eliminate them by a combination of education and 'naming and shaming', despite increasing evidence that relying on error-free performance is bound to fail.

The importance of dependable local delivery

No nationally based system, whether professionally or managerially led, is likely to succeed unless it can be delivered by effective local systems. Furthermore, as has been seen in the development of guidelines and protocols and in the attempt to introduce mandatory audit, the 'top-down' approach with systems being imposed on the local community by some central regulator is less effective than one in which local initiative is encouraged and where local groups develop a sense of ownership of the systems within a general overall national structure. In the past the ability of local groups to work together to ensure the delivery of high quality care, to work towards continuing development and to deal effectively with poor performance has been the weakest link in the quality assurance chain, both professionally and managerially. Whilst most individuals appear to take their responsibilities for continuing self-improvement seriously, the culture has seldom been conducive to effective local quality assurance within teams. This is no less true within anaesthetic departments than in other areas of clinical practice, despite the facts that anaesthetists are often prepared to take on much wider responsibilities within their local health-care system than others, and that many anaesthetic departments are well organised and cohesive. One of the main problems is the increasingly litigious, complaint oriented 'name and shame' environment in which most anaesthetists work. Whilst Government documents in recent years have emphasised the need for a blame-free culture, there is, as yet, little evidence of its existence. The Royal College of Anaesthetists has had serious concerns over its ability to maintain the confidentiality of its critical incident-reporting scheme, which is essential if it is to fulfil its proposed function of improving patient care. The establishment of the National Patient Survey Agency is to be welcomed as this Government approved agency plans to develop a completely confidential national critical incident-reporting scheme that will seek ways to guarantee that information would remain solely within the agency. Time will tell whether this desirable goal is achievable.

The concept of 'whistle-blowing' itself implies an inability of those with concerns about a colleague's performance to be able to address them constructively with the individual concerned without some official third party being called in. The 'three wise men' scheme has largely been discredited, and those with suspicions about a colleague's performance are often genuinely confused about what action to take. There is an increasing awareness that natural loyalty to one's colleagues must not be allowed to threaten patient safety, but people are sometimes genuinely unsure who they can turn to for help and advice about whether it is necessary to invoke formal disciplinary procedures. The 'three wise men' scheme was often excessively confidential, and its performance was seldom subject to audit. Anecdotal reports suggest that its effectiveness was extremely variable between individual Trusts and sometimes even within Trusts. There appears to be a need for an alternative local advisory system that, whilst preserving confidentiality when necessary, is more openly transparent and accountable than the 'three wise men' scheme. In one institution such a scheme is being piloted by the medical staff. A Professional Standards Advisory Committee has been established, composed of a group of doctors elected by their peers together with an appointed non-medical member, which provides a confidential advisory service for anyone with concerns about the conduct, health or performance of a doctor. Its terms of reference make it clear that confidentiality may have to broken in the interest of patient safety, though in practice ways can usually be found of avoiding this. The medical members of the committee are fully aware of their professional responsibility to the GMC to ensure that any patient safety issue of which they are made aware is effectively dealt with. Such schemes, however, are only likely to be successful if concerns are brought to them at an early stage so that problems can be addressed before they become serious.

In 1999, the UK Government announced new measures to protect 'whistle-blowers' and enable employees to raise concerns about NHS malpractice without being branded as troublemakers or damaging their career prospects[12]. Under the new guidelines Trusts are expected to:

- designate a senior manager to deal with employees' concerns and protect whistle-blowers
- have in place local policies and procedures and set out minimum requirements
- issue guidance to all staff so they know how to speak up against malpractice
- provide whistle-blowers with adequate protection against victimisation
- prohibit 'gagging' clauses in contracts.

Revalidation

It is perhaps surprising that, despite all the initiatives outlined above and the fact that the UK is seen internationally to have one of the best regulated medical professions in the world, criticism of our professionally led regulatory system continues to receive widespread media coverage. One justifiable concern arises from the fact that the GMC relies on reporting of allegedly deficient doctors either by individual patients or by local colleagues. This system has sometimes allowed seriously deficient doctors to practise for considerable periods of time whilst only their local colleagues were aware of their deficiencies. In February 1999, the GMC decided that all doctors would, in future, be required to demonstrate on a regular basis that they are up-to-date and fit to practice in their chosen field. Continuing medical registration would be linked with this demonstration in a practice now widely referred to as revalidation. Members of the public are frequently surprised that a doctor whose name is currently included in the medical register is not necessarily fit to practice. At present, entry in the register only indicates that at some time in the past the doctor satisfied the GMC's requirements for entry to the register, and has not subsequently been removed from it for disciplinary reasons. Revalidation will ensure that all doctors on the register are subject to continuing review of their performance.

It has been agreed that every five years doctors will be required to provide evidence of their fitness to practice, which must cover all areas of *GMP* as described above. It will be the doctor's responsibility to provide appropriate evidence, which will be reviewed by a panel of three GMC appointed and trained assessors, one of whom will be non-medical.

Revalidation will be a continuous process, during which doctors will be expected to have been subject to annual appraisal (Fig. 3.2). Following agreement between the Central Consultants and Specialists Committee of the British Medical Association (BMA) and the Department of Health (DOH), a proposal was agreed whereby appraisal would become mandatory for all consultants in the NHS, and standardised documentation was released for this purpose by the DOH[13]. For those working within the NHS, the mandatory annual appraisal scheme is likely to form the corner stone of revalidation. The GMC has embarked on a detailed pilot exercise to examine the quality of the link between the outputs of appraisal systems and the information needs for the purposes of revalidation. They have concluded that:

- The description of a doctor's current medical activities included within the appraisal documentation can give sufficient insight into the doctor's practice for revalidation.
- Robust underpinning evidence within the appraisal documentation, across the headings of Good Medical Practice, can give a clear insight into the doctor's performance and can be adequate for revalidation purposes.

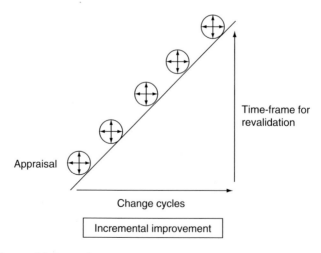

Figure 3.2. The revalidation cycle.

- When the appraisal documentation is complete, and contains a summary that reflects a robust appraisal discussion, it can be adequate for the purposes of revalidation without reference to the underpinning evidence.

Although appraisal is largely intended to be a formative process, it is a tribute to the close collaboration that has taken place between the medical profession and the Government that it has been designed to cover all aspects of good medical practice as required by the GMC. Much of the evidence that doctors will be required to produce for annual appraisal will, therefore, be usable in the revalidation exercise. It seems likely that this will include indicative information with respect to annual case or workload, up-to-date audit data with examples of how audit has changed the doctor's practice, and similar evidence from critical incident reporting, and any complaints received. Doctors will need to provide evidence of relevant continuing medical education and other professional development, but also evidence of satisfactory relationships with colleagues and patients. Those who teach or carry out research will be expected to include evidence of satisfactory performance in these areas, and it is likely that self-declarations of probity and health will also be required. The value of peer review is under consideration, but has been seen to be reliable in the United States[14]. The GMC is evaluating the use of peer review and patient satisfaction surveys as one way of providing part of the evidence required for revalidation. The joint working party of the Royal College and Association of Anaesthetists is building on the work it has already done in producing speciality-specific interpretations of *GMP* and has adapted its Personal Portfolio to help anaesthetists provide the speciality-specific evidence required to supplement Form 3 of the NHS appraisal documentation.

Despite natural initial concerns within the profession, there is now increasing confidence that this performance-based ongoing assessment will not only be fair and feasible but will also provide more valid evidence of a satisfactory standard of clinical practice than re-certification schemes based on tests of factual knowledge and skills alone. Failure to satisfy the revalidation committee will lead to referral to the GMC via its existing Fitness to Practice procedures, which contain built-in safeguard and appeal mechanisms. There will, however, be no extra hurdles or new threats facing doctors. For most, the scheme will involve little extra work on top of that required by existing continuing professional development programmes. On the other hand, there is now a real chance that the profession can give the public the assurance it requires that doctors remain capable and safe throughout their practising lives[15]. The benefits of this increased confidence between the public and the profession are obvious.

References

1. Irvine D. The performance of doctors I: professionalism and self-regulation in a changing world. Br Med J 1997; 314: 1540–2
2. General Medical Council. Good Medical Practice. London: GMC, 1995 (1st edn); 1998 (2nd edn); 2001 (3rd edn)
3. Royal College of Anaesthetists and Association of Anaesthetists of Great Britain and Ireland. Good Practice: A guide for departments of anaesthesia. London: RCA/AAGBI, 1998
4. NHS Executive. Clinical Governance: Quality in the New NHS. London: Department of Health, 1999

5. Williamson C. Representing patients. Bull Royal Coll Pathol 2001; 116: 26–7
6. Brennan TA, Leape LL, Laird N, et al. Incidence of adverse events and negligence in hospitalised patients: results of the Harvard Medical Practice Study I. N Engl J Med 1991; 324: 370–6
7. Wilson RM, Runciman WB, Gibberd RW, Harrison BT, Newby L, Hamilton JD. The quality in Australian health care study. Med J Austral 1995; 163: 458–71
8. Gopher D, Olin M, Donchin Y. The nature and causes of human errors in a medical intensive care unit. Presented at the 33rd meeting of the Human Factors Society. Denver CO, 1989
9. Reason J. Managing the Risks of Organisational Accidents. Aldershot: Ashgate, 1997
10. Perrow C. Normal accidents: living with high-risk technologies. New York: Basic Books, 1984
11. Department of Health. An organisation with a memory. Report of an expert group on learning from adverse events in the NHS. London: Department of Health, 2000
12. Department of Health. The Public Interest Disclosure Act 1998: Whistleblowing in the NHS. HSC 1999/198. London: Department of Health, 1999
13. Department of Health. NHS Appraisal for Consultants. 2001. Obtainable at *www.doh.gov.uk/nhsexec/consultantappraisal*
14. Ramsey PG, Wenrich MD, Carline JD, Inui TS, Larson EB, LoGerfo JP. Use of peer ratings to evaluate physician performance. JAMA 1993; 269: 1655–82
15. Irvine D. The performance of doctors. II: maintaining good practice, protecting patients from poor performance. Br Med J 1997; 314: 1613–17

Further Reading

Department of Health. A First Class Service: Quality in the New NHS. London: Department of Health, 1998
Hatch DJ. Revalidation, poor performance and clinical governance. In: Advancing Clinical Governance (M Lugon, J Secker-Walker, eds.) London: RSM Press, 2001: 149–61
Leape LL. Error in Medicine. JAMA 1994; 272: 1851–7
Reason J. Human Error. Cambridge University Press, 1990
Rosethal MM. The Incompetent Doctor: Behind Closed Doors. Buckingham PA: Open University Press, 1995

Confidentiality, Anaesthesia and Intensive Care $\qquad$ 4

Catherine Hale

Introduction

The requirement to protect patient confidentiality is the cornerstone of the doctor–patient relationship. Confidentiality has consistently formed a substantial part of the ethical codes of all health-care professionals. It is generally believed that the doctrine of confidentiality stems from the clinician's need to receive information that patients would normally keep secret or unsaid. Patients consciously make the decision to divulge sensitive and personal information where they have the confidence that the information they provide will remain confidential to their carers. The obligation of confidentiality within the role of clinician is examined below (see pp. 48, Should the obligation of confidentiality be an absolute or relative requirement?)

Part of the concept of confidentiality is the notion that patients have a right to control access to their own personal information. In other words, they have a right to privacy. As an indication of its importance, the right of privacy is now specifically recognised and protected by the *Human Rights Act 1998*. This piece of legislation incorporated the *European Convention on Human Rights* into domestic UK law and, therefore, governs the actions of employees of the NHS. *The Human Rights Act 1998* highlights that the obligation of doctors to maintain patient confidentiality extends far beyond the professional guidelines of the General Medical Council (GMC).

Any individual working with patients, in any circumstances, has a range of ethical, statutory and legal obligations in relation to confidentiality. In addition to the *Human Rights Act 1998*, certain Acts of Parliament specifically legislate on patient confidentiality. Similarly, under common law, an unauthorised disclosure of confidential information may lead to a case being pursued in court, for what is legally known as the 'equitable remedy of breach of confidence'.

The third sections of this chapter examines the legal obligation of confidentiality at common law (see pp. 51), including discussion of remedies for breach of confidence. The fourth section (see pp.57, Statutory requirements and exceptions to confidentiality) provides an analysis of the protection of patient confidentiality accorded by statute, including the *Human Rights Act 1998* and those situations in which statute requires that confidence to be broken.

In law, the protection given to patient information is not absolute. In some situations health-care professionals may be required to break confidentiality by statute, court order or at common law. In addition, there is a legal 'no-man's land' relating to information that (while generally protected by the obligation of confidentiality) may be disclosed in certain situations if it is in the public interest to do so. Perversely, the question of whether to disclose confidential information may arise more often today because modern clinicians often know more about their patients than their historical counterparts. Therefore, the fifth section, When ordered by the court (pp. 58), specifically considers disclosure of information and legal proceedings.

While patients have some means of redress where information is disclosed without their consent, until very recently they frequently faced considerable problems in obtaining access to their own health-care records. This position has gradually altered due to legislative changes, most recently, by the introduction of the *Data Protection Act 1998*. Nevertheless, patients still do not have an absolute right to access all of their records; access can be restricted if it is deemed not to be in the patient's best interests (see pp. 59, Patient access to health records).

In clinical practice, protecting patient confidentiality may give rise to a range of difficult moral and legal dilemmas. Within the environmental constraints of a public Intensive Care Unit (ICU), specific difficulties and problems may arise (see pp. 61, Specific problems in ICU in relation to patient confidentiality). For example, the way in which ICU is organised often means that private information is on public display. In addition, advances in technology mean that increasingly more is knowable and recorded about patients. Many different health-care practitioners, who work together in a multi-disciplinary team, care for patients who enter ICU. Therefore, many people have access to patient records, making confidentiality more difficult. Also, many patients who enter ICU may not be conscious and, therefore, may be unable to consent to the passing of their personal information. Given its focus on confidentiality in the context of ICU, this chapter will examine all of the above issues.

Should the obligation of confidentiality be an absolute or relative requirement?

The obligation of confidence is a dependent and integral part of the relationship of trust between doctor and patient. The first key question is whether the obligation of confidence is an absolute or a relative ethical concept?

From where does the obligation of confidence originate? If the source is the Hippocratic Oath, the obligation is a relative one only for the oath restricts disclosure only to that 'which *ought* not to be noised abroad'. It would seem, however, that as the obligation has evolved it has metamorphosed into an absolute duty: 'I will respect the secrets which are confided in me, even after the patient has died'[1].

The concept of an absolute duty is easier to pronounce, understand and assimilate. Expressed in Kantian terms, confidences should always be kept, regardless of the outcome. The health-care professional then needs only to know and concern themselves with the single principle and value: patients' confidences should be kept; they have no need to concern themselves with competing values, considerations and circumstances. The principle of confidentiality is not to be contained or curtailed by other criteria and especially not by that of consequence.

In contrast, a relative duty is obviously more sensitive to the individuality of each particular set of circumstances, but it is so much more difficult to articulate, relay and comprehend. The duty of confidence is still there, but it contains a proviso: confidences should always be kept, unless there is a better reason not to keep that confidence. The ensuing result is a diffuse professional uncertainty in difficult cases about what is the right thing to do and which value should be given primacy. Where confidentiality is considered to be a relative duty, the individual health-care professional is isolated and left to select and extract the correct moral choice. Now that the concepts of 'relative' and 'absolute' confidentiality have been defined, we will now move onto a discussion of the arguments for and against each approach.

Confession or confidence?

To argue that the duty of confidentiality is absolute as Kottow does[2] is not to acknowledge the fundamental and essential difference between the absolutes of religious confession and the relativities of the law of confidence. For while there is some symmetry between confession and confidence (in that a confession is to save the immortal soul and a medical confidence is to save the mortal body), implicit in the notion of confession is the acknowledgement of wrong to a divine silence and not merely the imparting of secrets with trust to another. This difference has been obscured since the Enlightenment.

In the years prior to the Reformation, information given to a priest during the confessional was privileged from disclosure in a court of law[3]. After the Reformation the case of *Broad* v. *Pitt* revealed the ambivalence of the law to confession[4]. Best CJ is recorded stating: 'I for one will never compel a clergyman to disclose communications to him by a prisoner but if he chooses to disclose them I shall receive them in evidence.'

In modern times, the boundaries between religious confession and the law of confidence have been so blurred that there are calls for medical confidences to be absolute and religious confessions are no longer treated as legally privileged. These dissipated boundaries are located wherever the twin issues of communication of secrets and the realisation of mortality intersect. Nowhere is this more apparent than in an ICU, where critically ill people may provide highly sensitive information in confidence. This is analogous to religious confessions because the patient either believes the information is necessary to save their physical life – for example, they may divulge that they have taken illegal substances – or, when critically ill and facing the prospect of death, they may share information about some wrongdoing with a healthcare professional, as a way of relieving their conscience.

49

Confidentiality as a relative concept

These false boundary claims mean that those who call for medical confidences to be absolute are fundamentally confused about the history of the notion of confidence and confession. The real argument is about the relativist stance: confidences should always be kept, unless there is a better reason not to keep that confidence. The absolutists claim this is merely a lack of rules. However, this objection fails because it is clearly possible to have rules that have exceptions to them, as long as these exceptions are clearly laid out. For example, it is both a legal and an ethical rule that a patient's consent is obtained before treatment, unless the patient is unconscious and the treatment is urgent. As Hart puts it[5]:

> . . . to argue in this way is to ignore what rules are in any sphere of real life. It suggests that we are faced with the dilemma: 'Either rules are what they would be in the formalists' heaven and they bind as fetters bind; or there are no rules, only predicable decisions or patterns of behaviour. Yet surely this is a false dilemma. A rule that ends with the word 'unless' is still a rule.'

According to Hart's defence of relativism, the duty of medical confidentiality is normative and conditional. The relative duty of confidentiality fuses two concepts of conscience. The first is the morality of a collective conscience, which preserves patients' autonomy by keeping promises of confidentiality. The second concept is the individual moral conscience of the autonomous professional. The result is that where obligations to patients compete, the nature and extent of the obligation of confidentiality will be contingent as part of the role as health-care professional. In other words health-care professionals find themselves at the sharp end, deciding when confidentiality should be breached.

The health-care professional must, in a situation of conflicting obligations, establish what counts as a good reason for breaching what would ordinarily count as a rule to maintain patient confidentiality. 'This approach parallels ordinary moral decision-making, in which choice between conflicting obligations is left to the decision-making agent as a responsibility of the role; where moral dilemmas occurring within the role are part of the role itself'[6].

Whether to disclose sensitive information and thereby to breach the ethical duty of confidentiality, or to maintain confidentiality, is part of a health worker's role, and integral to the job. So the role of the health-care worker in maintaining the obligation of confidence is recognised by the legal system in a particular way, allowing good-faith judgements by health-care professionals in the resolution of dilemmas in matters of confidentiality. Simply because no absolute, predetermined guide of when to disclose can be created in advance, decisions have to be made in the context of the role and that individual patient. The advantage of this approach is that the roles of health-care professionals are tried and tested, and they have a durability that is not easily overridden, but they also have a cultural component that renders them properly open to continuing review by the very people who continue to perform the role: health-care professionals.

The legal obligation of confidentiality at common law

The law recognises the competing nature of obligations within the role of all health-care professionals, including those based in an ICU environment. As such the common law imposes an obligation where it would be 'unconscionable' for the doctor to disclose information but nevertheless allows 'conscionable' disclosures where there is a stronger public interest in disclosure. This principle was laid down in the so-called 'Spycatcher case'[7].

The basis of a legal cause of action

To establish a cause of action in equity that a doctor unconscionably disclosed information, a patient must, in the words of Megarry J[8], demonstrate three things:

> . . . First, the information itself, in the words of Lord Greene MR in *Saltman Engineeering Co Ltd* v. *Campbell Engineering Co Ltd (1948) [1963] 3 All ER 413 at 415*, must 'have the necessary quality of confidence about it.' Secondly, that information must have been imparted in circumstances importing an obligation of confidence. Thirdly, there must be an unauthorised use of that information to the detriment of the party communicating it . . .

Once these elements are satisfied, the burden lies on the defendant health-care professional to prove some justification for the disclosure.

Legal remedies

Remedies for breach of the duty of confidence tend to be limited. Injunctions prior to disclosure can restrain disclosures, but they have no role to play once the breach has taken place. Financial compensation in the form of damages is not usually available for the breach of medical confidences. If the information is untrue then the patient can obviously sue for defamation of character, but usually the problem is that the information is true! Generally, enforcement of the professional obligation of confidence rests with the GMC, and likewise any subsequent disciplinary action, although the courts are the final arbiters of the practitioner's legal duty of confidentiality. Nevertheless, although the GMC's guidelines do not have statutory authority, the courts have acknowledged them as valuable in establishing the breadth of the practitioner–patient relationship.

The common law boundaries of the duty of confidentiality

To other carers participating in care on a 'need to know' basis   The classical approach to medical confidentiality of a one-to-one doctor–patient relationship where the patient discloses confidences to their doctor, which their doctor then binds themselves not to reveal, is almost unrecognisable in the context of intensive care and anaesthetics. The notion of implied consent is used as a basis for disclosure to all of the health-care team where a patient is in the care of more than one person. In such a case, the patient may be assumed to consent to all medical and nursing members of the team being informed so as to properly to carry out their respective obligations. It is, of course, also assumed that members of the 'team' who receive the information receive it in confidence. However, as Lord Goff remarked in *Re F*[9], implied consent is 'artificial' and 'difficult to impute' where the patient is incompetent. Disclosure, whether to health professionals, relatives or others, must in this instance be justified on a different principle. In practice, a patient who enters intensive care will frequently be unaware of the extent to which they will be examined and treated by junior doctors, anaesthetists and surgeons, who will also have access to patients' records. An American consultant, Siegler, carried out a survey after one of his patients threatened to leave hospital unless he was told how many people had access to his medical records. Siegler was staggered to discover that at least 75 and possibly as many as 100 medical personnel had legitimate access to that patient's records[10]. This number would probably have been higher had the patient's treatment been in an ICU or a teaching hospital.

With the patient's consent   Although consent is often regarded as an exception to the obligation of confidence, in fact, it is not. It is merely the recognition by the patient that the doctor is no longer under an obligation to keep the confidence; it defeats the existence of obligation. The problem in ICU is that it is very often impossible to obtain the patient's consent because the patient is unconscious.

Teaching, research and clinical audit   Access to patient information may be required in the pursuit of medical research and when teaching health-care professionals, as well as in the maintenance of medical standards by clinical audit. The precise remit of when data can be accessed for these purposes is determined by a combination of sources including: the GMC, the Department of Health, and the common law.

The GMC appears to have three main principles[11]:

- anonymise the data where possible
- normally obtain the express (and informed) consent of the patient
- disclosure may be justified without such consent in some circumstances. For example, in research, disclosure may be justified in exceptional circumstances without consent with the agreement of the appropriate Research Ethics Committee.

It is important to notice that the GMC does not seem to contemplate use for teaching or clinical audit without the express consent if the information is not anonymised[11]. It has been decided by the courts that it is not a breach of confidence to disclose anonymised patient data[12].

The Department of Health advises that written patient notices should be displayed informing patients why information about them is collected and to whom this information may be passed[13].

NHS and management purposes   There is a public interest in monitoring the efficient and appropriate use of public funds within the NHS. There is both statutory backing for financial auditors to access patient information (*National Health Service Act 1977*) and recognition of the need to appropriately monitor the use of public monies spent on health by the European Court of Human Rights. The European Court of Human Rights relied on art. 8(2) of the Convention in *MS v. Sweden*[14], finding that disclosure to monitor proper use of public funds was necessary for 'the economic well-being of the country'.

Disclosure in the public interest   There is a well-established and well-understood legal and ethical presumption in favour of confidentiality. Compelling reasons are, therefore, necessary in order to justify disclosure by a health-care professional of information acquired in practice. What constitutes 'a better reason', however, is not as well understood and health-care professionals encounter moral and ethical dilemmas as discussed above. Some reasons for disclosure palpably fail the better reason test: gossip with friends or colleagues, publication for public consumption, or to discuss the case of an identifiable or identified patient in publications without their consent.

Cases of child abuse, or where someone is infected with a communicable and potentially fatal disease, appear, however, to provide better reasons in order to justify disclosure. It is here, though, that the primary justification for medical confidentiality hits hardest because such patients are much less likely to seek appropriate medical assistance if they know that there is a real chance of being publicly revealed and their secrets defiled. Additionally, for Kottow[2] excusing breaches of confidence on grounds of superior moral values is unfair because it introduces an arbitrariness and ethical unreliability into the medical context. Health-care professionals are justifiably reluctant to disclose information, which may be in the public interest to disclose.

As discussed above, the courts recognise the competing nature of obligations within the role of health-care professionals. Therefore, the common law imposes an obligation of confidence on the doctor not to disclose information but, nevertheless, allows exceptional disclosures where there is a stronger public interest in disclosure, as in the case of *W* v. *Egdell*[15]. W had been detained in a secure hospital without limit of time, after successfully pleading the partial defence of diminished responsibility to a charge of murder, having killed five people and wounded another two. Eight years after he was sentenced, his medical officer at the hospital considered that W's medical condition had improved, and it was such that he could be transferred from the hospital to a regional secure unit. W decided to apply to a Mental Health Review Tribunal for discharge or transfer to a less secure unit. W's solicitors, in an attempt to obtain a report in support of the application, instructed Egdell, a consultant psychiatrist. Egdell formed the opinion that W was suffering from a paranoid psychosis and possibly had a psychopathic deviant personality and, therefore, strongly opposed W's application for discharge and expressed concern at a possible transfer. After receiving Dr. Egdell's report, W's solicitors unsurprisingly decided to withdraw the application to the tribunal. Dr Egdell, on finding that the report had not been sent to the hospital, took it upon himself to send a copy to the hospital director and agreed that a copy should be sent to the Home Office. W's solicitors argued that as there was a doctor–patient relationship between Egdell and W, and that Egdell was, therefore, bound by the obligation of confidentiality and should not have disclosed the report to anyone other than W or his representatives.

The Court of Appeal offered the following analysis:

> . . . there are two competing public interests . . . of course W has a private interest but the duty of confidence owed to him is based on the broader ground of public interest.

These competing interests are that the law should recognise professional duties of confidence and the public interest requires that patients should speak freely, openly and without fear to their doctors. Competing against this, Bingham LJ states that a doctor:

> . . . who becomes aware, even in the course of a confidential relationship, of information which leads him, in the exercise of what the court considers a sound professional judgment, to fear that . . . decisions may be made on the basis of inadequate information and with a real risk of consequent danger to the public is entitled to take such steps as are reasonable in all the circumstances to communicate the grounds of his concern to the responsible authorities . . .

Thus the competing public interests are identified as the preservation of the confidentiality of the doctor–patient relationship weighed in the balance against the wider public safety. Given the court's acceptance of the fact that confidence may be breached in the public interest, what are the factors that limit the extent to which information may be disclosed? The legal ruling of Egdell reveals that there are three.

First, as Bingham LJ makes clear, the disclosure may be made only to those whom it is necessary to tell so as to protect the public interest. Bingham LJ:

> He could not lawfully sell the contents of his report to a newspaper, as the judge held. Nor could he, without a breach of the law as well as professional etiquette, discuss the case in a learned article or in his memoirs or in gossiping with friends, unless he took appropriate steps to conceal the identity of W.

Secondly, to justify disclosure the risk must be 'real' as opposed to fanciful[15]. Thirdly, the risk in Egdell was to physical safety of members of the public (per Stephen brown P at 846 and Bingham LJ at 853QY3). It can be argued that the court only contemplated disclosure where there is a risk involving the danger of physical harm, given the emphasis placed on this aspect of the case by all the judges. The GMC's guidance appears to contemplate a slightly wider scope[11], stating that:

> Disclosure of personal information without consent may be justified where a failure to do so may expose the patient or others to a risk of death or serious harm . . . [although it is] wise to seek advice from professional association or medical defence union.

Confidentiality maintained in the public interest

In the case of *X* v. *Y*[16], freedom of the press was pleaded as a reason why a newspaper might print the breach of confidence that two practising general practitioners (GPs) were diagnosed as having contracted human immunodeficiency virus (HIV). Press freedom was, and is, protected by article 10 of the *European Convention on Human Rights* and is now given domestic protection by the *Human Rights Act 1998*. Free speech will only be restricted where the requirements of confidentiality are particularly strong. In *X* v. *Y*, the two doctors having contracted HIV underwent counselling at a local hospital to help them come to terms with the fact that they were HIV positive and to explore necessary precautions to avoid transmitting the condition to others. The GPs, after counselling, decided to continue with their medical practice. An employee of the health authority passed the medical records of these doctors to a journalist, who used them as a basis for an article in a tabloid newspaper. The health authority sought an injunction to prevent publication. The court weighed the public interest in retaining the confidentiality of acquired immune deficiency (AIDS) related information against the public interest of freedom of the press. The public interest in confidentiality was said to substantially outweigh the interest of press publication for three reasons. First, the doctors, as patients, ought to have their confidentiality preserved, with the hope of securing wider public health by encouraging patients with the virus to come forward for treatment. Second, hospital records should remain confidential, and third, employees should not disclose confidential information obtained in the course of their employment.

Is a health professional ever under a duty to disclose information?

It is arguably better to disclose to third parties who might be at risk as a result of the patient's actions, rather than authorities, especially as we do not inform the world at large but a single person only. The North American case of *Tarasoff* v. *Regents of the University California*[17] examined the notion of a health-care practitioner's liability for failing to disclose confidential information and warn a third party of his patient's intentions. In this case, the patient informed his therapist of an intention to kill a third party who, although not named, was clearly a girl with whom the patient had become infatuated. The patient did indeed murder the young woman two months later, in spite of attempts by the therapist to thwart such acts of violence. The parents of the murdered girl sued on the basis of the therapist's breach of duty to warn her of the likely danger. It was held that:

> A psychotherapist treating a mentally ill patient . . . bears a duty to use reasonable care to give threatened parties such warning as are essential to their foreseeable danger arising from the patient's condition or treatment.

There is no UK case law on this type of third party liability, as yet! So it is not clear whether the UK courts would impose civil liability on a doctor in a Tarasoff-type situation. It is unlikely that they would, but the more foreseeable and likely the harm, the more likely a court would be to consider that a doctor has a duty to breach confidence and warn a third party.

55

For clinicians in anaesthetics and intensive care, HIV infection, and the disease AIDS, has revealed the most substantial tension between the duty to the individual patient and the duty to protect others. How far should a doctor go in attempting to protect or notify others about HIV risk from their patient? Many clinicians are very uncomfortable with knowing that an HIV-positive patient may have infected others whom the patient is unwilling to inform. After attempting to influence the patient's behaviour or willingness to disclose his or her HIV status, the clinician may be left either unable to act further because of confidentiality, or feeling obliged to breach confidentiality to protect the third party. GMC guidance allows either, so long as the clinician is able to justify his or her actions. Each case must be judged on its particulars, so where a patient is HIV positive or has AIDS and withholds consent re disclosure, the practitioner may have a professional duty to ensure that any (identifiable) sexual partner is informed. Nevertheless, if patients perceive that a doctor will breach confidentiality to protect others, such information may no longer be forthcoming. The clinician must, therefore, determine the exact nature of the duty of confidentiality within the framework of their role with that particular patient.

Secrets of the dead

Unfortunately, despite the success of advances in technology patients do die in ICU and health-care professionals need to be able to answer the question: 'what effect does the death of a patient have on the common law obligation of confidence?' The traditional ethical principle is stated by the GMC as follows[11]:

> You still have an obligation to keep personal information confidential after a patient dies. The extent to which confidential information may be disclosed after a patient's death will depend on the circumstances. These include the nature of the information, whether that information is already public knowledge or can be anonymised and the intended use to which the information will be put. You should also consider whether, and if so to what extent, the disclosure of information may cause distress to, or be of benefit to, the patient's partner or family . . .

Death does not appear to cancel the obligation of confidentiality as illustrated by the following two cases, which involve doctors who published details of their deceased patients' medical information without their patients' consent. After Sir Winston Churchill died, his physician Lord Moran wrote a book entitled *Churchill: The Struggle for Survival (1944–1965)*; which revealed that in the latter years of Churchill's premiership he suffered a dramatic decline in health. Publication of the book led to great debate, and the author attracted critical comment from his colleagues in the medical profession. Likewise in 1983 the *British Medical Journal* published an obituary of Gladwin Buttle, who had largely been responsible for the use of blood transfusions on a large scale during the Second World War. The obituary contained Buttle's medical opinion after he had treated a General Wingate, who had cut his own throat. The general opinion at the time was that General Wingate was insane, but Buttle's notes revealed that the General's blood was swimming with malarial parasites. The editor of the *British Medical Journal* received a letter from the GMC, which informed him that, although the details in the obituary were by no means disparaging towards the General, the disclosure was nevertheless in breach of confidence[18]. However, it may be possible to advance an argument in favour of Buttle's actions because, as the GMC conceded, it was arguably in the patient's interests to disclose this information, even without consent (for consent would have be impossible to obtain). Buttle may well have considered it better for General Wingate's reputation that he was not thought to be insane at the time of his death.

Incompetent patients, unconsciousness and confidentiality

Does the fact that the patient lacks capacity (as so often is the case in ICU due to unconsciousness) mean that there is no common law obligation of confidentiality? There is an obligation of confidence implied as a consequence of any doctor–patient relationship, including where the patient is incompetent. However, there is no decided authority as to whether information concerning an incompetent adult can be disclosed, for example, to their relatives. It would seem likely that the courts would adopt the same test as the House of Lords did in *F* v. *West Berkshire Health Authority*[19], so that disclosure can take place if those treating the patient believe that it is necessary in the best interests of the patient. Adoption of this approach requires doctors to exercise considerable discretion. It is suggested that the best interests of the patient would require that confidential information should only be disclosed on a 'need to know' basis.

Statutory requirements and exceptions to confidentiality

Statutory requirements to maintain confidentiality

Until the *Human Rights Act 1998*, there was no general statutory protection that medical information should be kept confidential. However, certain statutory provisions require particular types of health information to be kept confidential. It is unsurprising that the statutory protection that existed prior to the *Human Rights Act 1998* related, and still relates, to areas of health-care practice widely considered to be of a particularly sensitive nature, such as infertility treatment or treatment for venereal disease.

Human Rights Act 1998

The importance of confidentiality as a human right is protected by the *European Convention on Human Rights*, which, of course, is now incorporated into English law by the *Human Rights Act 1998*. The recent case *A Health Authority* v. *X & ORS*[20] recognised the two recent decisions of the European Court of

Human Rights in *Z* v. *Finland*[21] and *MS* v. *Sweden*[14], illustrating the application of article 8 of the convention, which provides for 'the right to respect for [an individual's] private and family life' (art. 8(1)). In the case of *A Health Authority* v. *X & ORS*, the court stated that there was a compelling pubic interest requiring the disclosure of medical records to a health authority investigating allegations that medical practitioners had breached their terms of service. However, disclosure of medical records to a public body was an interference with a patient's rights under article 8 of the *European Convention on Human Rights* and could only be justified where there were effective and adequate safeguards against abuse.

Statutory requirements to disclose confidential information

Some statutes expressly require that patient confidentiality should be broken. Information is generally required for the purposes of the investigation of crime or where disclosure is required on public health grounds. For example, the police may want disclosure of medical information from a patient's notes during a criminal investigation. Disclosure is regulated in these circumstances by the *Police and Criminal Evidence Act 1984*, which was amended during its passage through Parliament to take account of the concerns expressed by the British Medical Association (BMA) that the reform of police powers rendered patient information unjustifiably vulnerable to access. Therefore, those seeking access to such records must now obtain a warrant from a circuit judge. Other statutes requiring information to be notified include the following: *Human Organ Transplants Act 1989, Abortion Act 1967, Public Health (Control of Disease) Act 1984, Prevention of Terrorism Act 2000* and the *Road Traffic Act 1988*.

When ordered by the court

The English courts have, in modern times, consistently rejected suggestions that a privilege be introduced allowing doctors to refuse to disclose confidential health information when requested by a court. Medical information may, however, be withheld from disclosure prior to or during a trial if protected by legal professional privilege. Legal professional privilege protects information passed between lawyer and client.

However, health-care professionals must disclose where required to do so by force of law either by way of a judicial decision or under statutory rule. At law, confidential communications between physicians and patients receive no protection against disclosure in legal proceedings, despite the fact that disclosures of the very same confidential information when occurring outside the courtroom may be viewed as unethical and a breach of confidence.

In the *Duchess of Kingston's Case*[22], the court refused to recognise the physician–patient privilege. Mr Hawkins, a physician who had attended the defendant (who had been accused of bigamy) and her alleged husband, was asked: 'Do you know from the parties of any marriage between them?' Lord Chief Justice Mansfield stated:

> If a surgeon was voluntarily to reveal these secrets, to be sure he would be guilty of a breach of honour and a grave indiscretion but to give that information in a court of justice which by the law of the land he is bound to do will never be imputed to him as an indiscretion whatever.

This, therefore, confirms that the law recognises and upholds a relative, not an absolute, duty of confidentiality. A doctor compelled to provide information to a court may well risk punishment for contempt of court by refusing to break a patient's confidence and make disclosure. A pertinent example for ICU practitioners who treat patients who have been involved in road traffic accidents is that of *Hunter* v. *Mann*[23], whereby a doctor treating emergency patients involved in a car accident refused to disclose their identity to the police, on the basis of confidences placed in him. This justification did not prevent his prosecution in the Magistrates' Court under a section of the *Road Traffic Act 1972*, which demands that 'any person . . . shall be required . . . to give any information which it is in his power to give and may lead to the identification of the driver.' He appealed against this decision on the basis that, as the information was given in confidence, it was never 'in his power' to make disclosure. His appeal failed, clearly illustrating that the law recognises no professional privilege not to disclose confidences to a court, other than that of the legal profession.

Patient access to health records

For many years the medical profession resisted calls for patients to be given rights of access to their medical records. However, the opposing view, that access can be regarded as part of recognising a patient's autonomy and may assist them in decision-making has gradually gained primacy, and this is given statutory protection through the *Data Protection Act 1998*. Nevertheless, this statutory right is not absolute and disclosure can still be withheld if the information would be harmful to the patient's mental or physical health.

Prior to the *Data Protection Act 1998*, patients' access to their own medical records was governed by two Acts of Parliament, namely the *Data Protection Act 1984* and the *Access to Health Records Act 1990*. The former covered electronically stored records and the latter manually written records created after November 1991. The *Data Protection Act 1984* and *Access to Health Records Act 1990* have now been largely replaced by the *Protection Act 1998*, which gives effect to the European Directive on Personal Data (OJ L281). The only remaining remit of the *Access to Health Records Act 1990* is pertaining to patients who are deceased. Therefore, all health records for current patients, both electronic and manual, are now covered by the 1998 Act (s1(1)), regardless of when they were created, since the Act is, unusually, retrospective.

Section 7 of the *Data Protection Act 1998* confers a right of access upon an individual (the 'data subject') to certain information from a 'data controller'. The data controller is required to supply the information 'promptly'. In order to trigger the data controller's obligation to supply the information, the following must apply:

- there must be a request in writing to supply information
- the data controller must receive a fee not exceeding the prescribed maximum (usually £10)
- the data controller must be supplied with 'such information as he may reasonably require in order to satisfy himself as to the identity of the person making the request and to locate the information which the person seeks'.

Subject to certain limitations the data controller must supply the following information:

- whether the personal data, of which the individual is the subject, are being processed by or on behalf of the data controller
- a description of the data, the purposes for which it is being processed and the recipients (or classes of recipients) to whom it may be disclosed
- if required by the data subject, where possible and which would not involve disproportionate effort, a copy in a permanent and intelligible form of the information held including the source of the data – and this may include an explanation of any terms used
- the logic of any process of automated data processing applied to the data.

However, access to health records is limited by the *Data Protection* (subject access modification) *(Health) Order 2000* (SI 2000, No. 413), which creates an exemption from access under section 7. The exemption arises if the disclosure of medical records would be likely to cause serious harm to the physical or mental health or condition of the data subject or any other person. Critically ill patients in ICU may find that they fall within this exemption if they wish to see their clinical records, as the information is likely to contain information that their life was and or is still in danger. The psychological effects of such information at best would be quite profound and may well be determined to be likely to be harmful to their physical and/or mental health.

If a doctor fails to comply with a request under section 7, the data subject may make an application to the court for access under section 7(9). The court can order the data controller to comply with the request. The patient may also recover compensation for any 'damage' suffered as a result of the doctor's failure to comply with the request (section 13), which may include financial or psychiatric injury. However, compensation for 'distress' alone is not recoverable under section 13. On application by the data subject, section 14 also gives a court power to order the data controller to 'rectify, block, erase or destroy' data which is 'inaccurate'.

The *Data Protection Act 1998* is specifically concerned with regulating the 'processing' of 'personal data' of 'data subjects' (patients) by 'data controllers' (s1(1)). Within the NHS, health service bodies will be 'data controllers' but individual doctors, may also be such. 'Processing' is given a very wide scope, and it includes virtually anything that is done with the personal data, such as obtaining, storing and using it in any way including disclosing it. 'Personal data' is also given a wide definition in section 191 of the 1998 Act. It includes expressions of opinion about the individual or statements of intention in relation to that individual. It is, however, restricted in two ways: it must relate to a 'living individual', and it must be information that identifies that individual or which may make the individual identifiable from other data or other information in, or likely to come into, the possession of the data controller. Therefore, the Act does not apply to information held about dead persons or where the information is adequately anonymised.

The *Access to Health Records Act 1990* is the legislation that covers information held about the deceased. Where the patient has died, an application may be made by the patient's personal representative or any person who may have a claim arising out of the patient's death. However, access may be excluded where the deceased has requested that they did not want access to be given on such an application. Access may also be excluded to any part of the record to the extent that the disclosure of the information is, in the opinion of the record holder, likely to cause serious harm to an individual (whether the applicant or someone else) or would reveal information about, or provided by, someone other than the patient unless he or she has consented or where that person is a health professional. The right of access is also restricted to records that came into existence on, or after, 1 November 1991.

Specific problems in ICUs in relation to patient confidentiality

The typical open-plan layout of an ICU – and the type of technologies used – ensures that patients and their monitors are clearly visible at all times to detect any signs of deterioration or improvement in patients' health. The downside is that there is a large amount of patient data routinely on show and observable by anyone walking past a patient's bedside. This seems like a clear dilemma: which should take precedence, patient safety or confidentiality? The dilemma seems to have been clearly resolved in favour of patient safety. However, because the dilemma seems to have been clearly resolved, this has arguably lead to complacency on the part of health-care workers and managers. Private information is routinely on display and discussed, without questioning whether that particular information needs to be shared so openly in order to deliver optimum patient care.

The very often forgotten questions, 'Does the information need to be displayed? How should the information be recorded? Whom should it be shared with?' are essential questions that need to be satisfactorily answered to ensure the ethical care of patients. Advances in medical technology mean we know more about patients in medical observable terms than we have ever known. We are, therefore, able to record more information about patients than we have ever recorded before. Technology is also beginning to allow us to record patient information in new computerised ways.

Therefore, advances in technology will continue the trend of making more information about patients receiving this type of care available and recordable, with the result that legal and ethical dilemmas are likely to increase rather than decrease in the foreseeable future.

Patient care in intensive care and anaesthetics is more complex than in any other discipline. The patient is cared for not by one or a small number of individuals but by many different health-care practitioners over any given 24-hour period. All of these health-care professionals are essential members of the multidisciplinary team and, as such, they have legitimate access to the patient's records. However, the more people who have access to patient records, the more difficult it is to think of patient records as being confidential. Nevertheless, professional and ethical guidelines are simultaneously enforcing the need to combat this attitude, and the introduction of the *Human Rights Act 1998* makes it clear that the both the public and parliament wish this information to be kept confidential.

Due to the innovations of intensive care and anaesthetics, patients are now surviving major traumas, illnesses and operations. This almost invariably means that the patient is unconscious at some stage during their care. In fact, the majority of patients that are treated in an operating theatre and intensive care are unconscious. This means that patients are incapable at that time of giving consent for their confidentiality to be breached. Rather than this being a justification to breach confidentiality, it means that the ICU practitioner is probably under an even greater burden to protect vulnerable unconscious patients because they are unable to speak for themselves. Nevertheless, this duty is to be balanced against the need for the disclosure of a patient's prognosis to worried relatives. This can be justified as being in the best interests of the patient who generally would wish to alleviate their relative's anxiety.

Summary

The requirement to protect patient confidentiality remains the cornerstone of all health-care professional–patient relationships, including those within an ICU setting; it was examined above and determined to be a 'relative' rather than an 'absolute' concept. The range of ethical, statutory and common law obligations that are owed to patients in ICU, in relation to maintaining confidentiality were then discussed, followed by an examination of protection to patient confidentiality accorded by statute. The right of privacy is now specifically protected by the *Human Rights Act 1998*, which governs the actions of the NHS and its employees. However, in contrast, it was demonstrated that certain Acts of Parliament specifically legislate requiring a breach of patient confidentiality, usually on public health grounds.

It was also revealed that the situations in which health-care professionals may be required to break confidentiality are regulated by court order and common law as well as by statute. In addition, the parameters of the legal 'no-man's land' were discussed, where there is a discretion to breach patient confidentiality, if and only if it is in the public interest to do so. The recent regulations that now govern patients' access to their records were then discussed. Generally, patients now have a legally enforceable right to see their own health-care records. However, this is still not an absolute right, and access can be restricted if it is deemed not to be in the patient's best interests.

Finally, the specific difficulties and problems around patient confidentiality that arise in ICU were examined. It was argued that the way in which ICU is organised often means that private information is on public display. In addition, advances in technology have meant that, increasingly, more is known and recorded about patients. Also, the fact that many patients who enter ICU may not be conscious was specifically considered.

References

1. The World Medical Association Declaration of Geneva: Physician's Oath. 1948 (amended by the 22nd World Medical Assembly, Sydney, Australia, August 1968) WMA
2. Kottow M. Medical confidentiality: an intransigent and absolute obligation. J Med Ethics 1986; 12: 117–22
3. McHale J. Medical Confidentiality and Legal Privilege. Routledge Kegan Paul, 1993: 24
4. *Broad v. Pitt* (1828) 3 C & P 518
5. Hart H. The Concept of Laws. Clarendon Press, 1961
6. Tur R. Medical confidentiality and disclosure: moral conscience and legal constraints. J Appl Philosophy 1998; 15: 15–28
7. *Attorney-General v. Guardian Newspapers* (No 2) [1990] 1 AC 109
8. *Coco v. A N Clark (Engineers) Ltd* [1969] RPC 41
9. *Re F (Mental Patient: Sterilisation)* [1990] 2 AC 1
10. Siegler, M. Confidentiality in Medicine – A Decrepit Concept. N Engl J Med 1982; 307: 1518–21
11. General Medical Council. Confidentiality: Protecting and Providing Information. GMC, 2000
12. *R v. Department of Health, ex p Source Informatics Ltd* (1999) 52 BMLR 65 (CA)
13. Department of Health. Protection and Use of Patient Information DOH, 1996
14. *MS v. Sweden* (1997) 45 BMLR 133
15. *W v. Egdell* [1990] 1 All ER 835 (CA)
16. *X v. Y* [1988] 2 All ER 648
17. *Tarasoff v. Regents of the University California* 529 P 2d 55 (Cal 1974)
18. McHale J. Medical confidentiality and legal privilege. Routledge Kegan Paul, 1993: 72–3
19. *F v. West Berkshire Health Authority* [1989] 2 All ER 545
20. *A Health Authority v X & ORS* (2001) (Lawtel 10/05/01)
21. *Z v. Finland* (1997) 25 EHRR 371
22. *Duchess of Kingston's Case* (1776) 20 State T 355
23. *Hunter v. Mann* [1974] QB 767

Further Reading

Bennet R, Draper H, Frith L. Ignorance is bliss? HIV and moral duties and legal duties to forewarn. J Med Ethics 2000; 26: 9–15

Emson H. Confidentiality: a modified value. J Med Ethics 1988; 14: 87–90

Mahendra B. Medical disclosure and confidentiality. N Law J 2001; 151: 10

Warwick S. Vote for no confidence. J Med Ethics 1989; 15: 183–5

Cultural Relativism, Tolerance and Respect for Autonomy   **5**

Andrew Fagan

Introduction

This chapter provides a moral philosopher's examination of an increasingly common ethical problem for clinicians; namely, what is the ethical response to a patient who refuses to consent to potentially life-saving medical treatment on the grounds that such treatment will entail a significant violation of the fundamental values and beliefs of the cultural community of which the patient is a recognised member?

It is sometimes argued that there is a moral duty to respect the specific and varying cultural values and beliefs of all human beings on the grounds that membership of a given culture is essential for human well-being generally. The implications of the extension of such a duty to the provision of medical treatment are profound when the moral demand to fully respect a patient's professed cultural beliefs conflicts with the cultural ethos of medical treatment, its aims and methods of treatment. In such instances, clinicians are apparently confronted by an ethically fraught situation, in which respecting the culturally informed wishes of the patient may require them to refrain from pursuing medically beneficial treatment on the grounds that such treatment will require a fundamental violation of that patient's religious and cultural beliefs. It is clear that a requirement to respect cultural and religious beliefs even, and especially, when these place medically avoidable constraints upon treatment raises some deeply problematic issues, which demand careful consideration.

This chapter aims to do precisely that: beginning with a brief survey of actual and potential examples of such conflict and consideration of their sociological origins; then moving on to consider the ethical issues raised; and concluding with an assessment of the prospects for resolving such conflict.

Multicultural medicine?

Complex societies, such as the United Kingdom and the United States, are increasingly multicultural in character. Within many of the large urban conurbations of both countries one can find a veritable Babel of immigrant native languages spoken, designating the existence of a similarly diverse array of cultural communities that have survived, and even thrived, despite geographical dislocation. While the implications of multiculturalism for the formulation of democratically legitimate political constitutions have been consistently analysed and discussed within the academic community generally[1-3], relatively little attention has been paid to the extent to which multiculturalism may affect the provision of medical treatment and the fundamental ethical principles that guide medical practice. This lack of attention to the possible effects of cultural diversity upon the principles and working practices of clinicians appears to support those who have consistently criticised biomedicine for ignoring the importance of culture, generally, in the successful provision of medical treatment[4]. Critics such as Helman[4] present biomedicine's commitment to a physiologically reductivist model of disease as largely excluding the possibility of fully appreciating the extent to which a given patient's subjective understanding of the nature and causes of his or her ailment can be influenced by the beliefs and values of the particular culture to which he or she belongs. A brief survey of the central tenets of a number of different contemporary cultural and religious belief systems will illustrate the extent to which such factors can influence a patient's understanding of the nature, causes and appropriate treatment of a given ailment.

The most frequently cited example is that of the Jehovah's Witnesses' prohibition of blood transfusion on the grounds that such a practice, even under conditions of medical necessity, constitutes an intolerable violation of that faith's fundamental religious beliefs. However, a sole dependence upon this particular example has been recently complicated by an unexpectedly reformist trend amongst some members of this religious community, which allows for a degree of individual discretion on this particular, formerly fundamental, religious tenet so that consenting to a blood transfusion is no longer absolutely prohibited amongst the followers of Jehovah.

Fortunately, for the purposes of this discussion, examples of less compromising cultural and religious communities are not hard to find.

The Christian Scientist church has long prohibited the use of vaccinations and inoculations amongst its members on the general grounds that any such medical intervention constitutes an unacceptable violation of that faith's central tenets. A conscientious commitment to such beliefs has resulted in the medically preventable death of at least one Christian Scientist[5]. In a more speculative vein, one may question how members of the Jain religious community, and even some of those who adhere to a strict vegetarian regimen, are likely to respond to the emergence and progressively extensive deployment of xenotransplantation, given both communities' prohibition against the use of animals in this fashion. Equally, the transplantation of animal organs into human bodies constitutes a clear violation of the human/non-human animal distinction which is itself sacred to the Judeo-Christian tradition generally.

Looking slightly further afield, whilst remaining with the topic of organ transplantation, it is also interesting to note that Japanese culture, generally, has long rejected the absence of brain activity as the sufficient criterion for determining when death occurs. This has been contrasted with western biomedicine's emphasis upon brain activity as the key criterion of the persistence of life. Ohnuki-Tierney[6], a medical anthropologist, argues that western culture generally differs from its Japanese counterpart on the central issue of the physiological location of personhood. She argues that the principal importance that western biomedicine accords to the brain, in this respect, is entirely consistent with a western philosophical perspective that views the exercise of reason as the key distinguishing characteristic of personhood. In contrast, Japanese conceptions of personhood may be described as more pluralist in character, identifying not one but several bodily organs as essential sites of personhood, including the liver and the stomach. While one may wish to take issue with such explanations, what is undeniable is that such beliefs have a profound effect upon Japanese perceptions of the ethical legitimacy of organ transplantation. Japan has some of the lowest rates of organ donation and organ transplantation in the developed world[6]. Amongst the more secularly minded inhabitants of Japan, this may be accounted for, in part, by a more rigorous measure of determining when the death of the would-be donor has occurred combined with a cultural reluctance to accept such symbolically significant organs as the stomach and the liver. In addition, Confucian religion generally insists that the successful rebirth of the soul is dependent upon retaining an intact body, in life and after death. Imagine how a follower of such beliefs is likely to respond to the prospect of becoming an organ donor after death! Clearly, amongst Japanese people generally, there exist powerful forces that serve to limit the medical use of organ transplantation as a means of preserving and prolonging life.

The examples cited above are not intended to be exhaustive, by any means. A fully comprehensive, empirical survey of the diverse cultural and religious communities found within many highly industrialised societies will reveal the full extent to which prospective patients' cultural beliefs may come into conflict with what clinicians will consider to be medically essential forms of treatment. In some instances, it will be possible to proceed with forms of alternative treatment that will be acceptable to both clinician and patient alike. While the medical prospects of those Jains and strict vegetarians requiring organ transplantation may be affected by a growing utilisation of xenotransplantation, the technique itself is not intended to wholly replace the use of human organs. A refusal to accept an animal's kidney on cultural, religious or moral grounds might extend the time a patient spends on dialysis, and thereby reduce the patient's chances of survival, but this need not, in itself, result in that patient's medically preventable death so long as the, albeit inadequate, supply of human organs remains. In a circumstance such as this, the clinician is not faced with a stark and immediate life-or-death scenario. However, such scenarios do arise. Individuals have refused to sanction medically essential treatment on the grounds that such treatment entails an unacceptable violation of the fundamental cultural and religious beliefs to which they adhere. In so doing these individuals are, in effect, prioritising their cultural and religious interests over their interests in health and well-being and, thereby, inadvertently perhaps, challenging the guiding presumption of western medicine that the prolongation of life and the restoration of health are of ultimate, incontrovertible value.

How then, ought clinicians ethically respond to those patients who refuse to consent to medical treatment on cultural grounds, even where such a decision, if respected, will result in a medically preventable death? What possible grounds can there be for clinicians suspending their commitment to the Hippocratic Oath? For answers to questions such as these it is necessary to address the ethical basis of the doctrine of multiculturalism and the call to respect other cultures' beliefs and practices.

Multiculturalism and respect for the other

The existence of a diverse collection of cultural and religious communities within a single society presents the provision of publicly funded and regulated services with a relatively new problem; namely, how to respond to the expressed wishes of those communities whose values and beliefs are found to be, in certain important respects, fundamentally incompatible with the principles upon which the provision of such services are based? Given the potential life-or-death consequences of medical treatment, clinicians may reasonably be thought of as peculiarly exposed to this particular problem. Hence, arguably, the question to which many clinicians require an answer is why a patient's culturally determined wishes should be respected at all? The answer to this particular question is complicated and multifaceted, but it begins with a consideration of the importance of culture to the development of our identity as individual human beings.

In recent years, the role that culture plays in the development and lives of human beings has been generally recognised. However, before one can properly begin to understand the arguments that philosophers have presented in support of this process, one must first understand what is meant by the term 'culture'. The medical practitioner and anthropologist C. G. Helman (p. 2)[4] defines culture as 'a set of guidelines (both explicit and implicit) that individuals inherit as members of a particular society, and that tell them how to view the world, how to experience it emotionally, and how to behave in it in relation to other people, to supernatural forces or gods, and to the natural environment'. Like many anthropologists and sociologists before him, Helman proceeds to argue that all human relations are conducted within a cultural context. Human behaviour is primarily acquired through socialisation in the values, beliefs and practices of one's family and the wider cultural community: human beings are, first and foremost, cultural animals. It is precisely this claim that provides the starting point for many of the philosophical arguments in support of multiculturalism.

In contrast to a well-established, primarily liberal philosophical tradition that presents individuals as self-constituting, ultimately self-reliant beings, philosophers such as Charles Taylor and Joseph Raz (to name but two) have increasingly come to emphasize the cultural basis of human identity and individual agency[3,7]. Both philosophers endorse the claim that human identity is constituted through culturally embedded relationships and practices. On this reading, our identities are acquired through our membership of, initially at least, one cultural community. Similarly, the acquisition of our personal identities is itself constituted through our identification with the varying values, beliefs and practices that are culturally constituted and determined. For philosophers such as Taylor and Raz, each individual's identity is shaped by, and is therefore ultimately dependent upon, the culture they have grown up within: we come to be the kinds of people we are as a result of the cultures we inhabit. As Taylor states, '(w)e become full human agents, capable of understanding ourselves, and hence of defining our identity, through our acquisition of rich human languages of expression' (p. 79)[8]. These languages of expression are themselves culturally embedded. In addition to their claim that all human identity has a cultural basis, both philosophers argue that, as culture-inhabiting beings, our exercise of choice always occurs within a general cultural setting, and that, further, the very objects of even our most significant choices are themselves culturally dependent. Thus, Raz argues that the choice to pursue a medical career is only possible within societies that both recognise the existence of such a specific profession and in which there exists the institutional infrastructure to support such a practice[9]. However, the general argument in support of multiculturalism goes further than the mere presentation of an empirical claim concerning the cultural basis of personal identity.

Following on from the initial claim that all human identity is culturally constituted, philosophical advocates of multiculturalism, such as Taylor and Raz, go on to argue that individual well-being is significantly dependent upon membership of a respected cultural community: one which is duly recognised within the wider society. The reason for this may be simply stated: because one's identity as an individual is constituted through one's relations with others and is prefigured, to a significant extent, by how others evaluate and perceive one as a member of a recognisable cultural community, the development of one's identity may be adversely affected by being associated with a cultural community that is the object of discrimination or prejudice. Multiculturalism is, in part, intended to rectify the systematic discrimination that many members of minority cultures testify to having experienced in their attempts to practice their own cultural beliefs and values within complex, industrialised societies. Clearly, if individual identity is culturally constituted, it follows that a given individual's well-being is dependent upon the general well-being of the culture to which he or she belongs. Advocates of multiculturalism typically go further in arguing that the state has a moral obligation to protect and promote its citizens' essential interests and that these interests include membership of a respected cultural community. Consequently, Taylor specifically requests of the state and individual citizens alike that due recognition and respect be extended to each individual's cultural community. He insists that 'due recognition is not just a courtesy we owe people. It is a vital human need' (p. 76)[8].

In addition to an argument concerning the value of culture to individual well-being, multiculturalists typically extend their argument to include support for what is widely termed the doctrine of value pluralism. Multiculturalists address their arguments to those societies in which there exist a number of diverse cultural and religious communities. Such societies may be described as normatively pluralist in character, in that there is likely to exist a number of differing, perhaps even incompatible, visions of how life ought to be led and differing opinions as to what practices and beliefs are genuinely valuable. Against those who argue that there is only one correct way to lead a morally valuable life, multiculturalists typically endorse the value pluralist argument that valuable human lives can be achieved in a diverse number of indeterminable ways: that there simply is no singly correct way to lead a morally valuable life. To this extent, multiculturalism may be thought of as continuing the long-established tradition within liberal political societies that, in theory at least, prohibits the state from attempting to dictate to its citizens how they ought to lead their lives[10]. Thus, in addition to the argument that presents the recognition of one's culture as a vital human need, advocates of multiculturalism also seek to justify their doctrine by the claim that the existence of a genuinely multicultural society may be understood as the realisation of the liberal doctrine of value pluralism under conditions of cultural diversity. Taken together, these two arguments constitute the basis of multiculturalism's philosophical legitimacy. But what, specifically, does the implementation of multicultural principles require of the state, and what initial implications might this have for the provision of medical treatment?

Both Taylor and Raz are unequivocal in their insistence that the withholding of recognition of the value of cultural communities can constitute a form of social and political oppression, in so far as the well-being and sense of self-worth of individual members of those communities is likely to be adversely affected as a result. However, neither philosopher is prepared to advocate extending equal recognition to all groups that designate themselves as 'cultures'. Rather, both insist that enjoying the political status that multiculturalism can confer upon cultures is dependent upon the satisfaction of certain conditions. Thus, Raz argues that 'multiculturalism requires a political society to recognise the equal standing of all the stable and viable cultural communities existing in that society' (p. 159)[3]. According to Raz, the crucial criteria for extending equal respect to any given culture are not determined by whether the values and beliefs of that culture conform to those espoused by the state, but depend rather upon the stability and viability of the particular culture in question. While they remain somewhat vague in character, Raz clearly intends the stability and viability conditions to serve as threshold criteria for determining which cultures ought to enjoy equal respect and recognition by the state. Such criteria might act to exclude the claims of newly established religious cults or political associations from claiming the status of a viable and stable culture.

It seems reasonable, however, to conclude that all of the cultural and religious groups I referred to earlier would have a legitimate claim to the state's respect and recognition, despite the apparent incompatibility between some of the central tenets of their cultural beliefs and values and the aims and aspirations of medical treatment. A state committed to the doctrine of multiculturalism is thereby morally obliged to extend equal respect and recognition to all those cultures that successfully satisfy the threshold criteria. This principally requires that the state formulate its political and legislative procedures in such a way as to be equally acceptable to all those cultures that fall under its jurisdiction. Similarly, it also requires that the state allocate the provision of public services and goods in a manner that accords equal respect and recognition to all the relevant legitimate cultures. What implications does this have for the ethical provision of medical treatment and, in particular, how would the realisation of this moral obligation affect the relationship between clinicians and those of their patients who refused to consent to treatment on cultural grounds?

Respecting the patient – autonomy and multiculturalism

The formulation of a coherent answer to the above questions must extend to include due consideration of the possibility of a recurring outcome that many medical practitioners may consider ethically unacceptable; namely, that fully respecting a patient's express refusal to consent to medical treatment on cultural grounds will require clinicians' violation of the Hippocratic Oath and the fundamental aims and aspirations of medical treatment. There can be little doubt that the full implementation of a multiculturalist policy within the health sector will result in an increase in the levels of medically preventable diseases and deaths. Is there any sense then, in which such a general policy can be successfully implemented in the provision of medical treatment? Or does it simply require too much of clinicians?

In large part, the bases of the possible ethical opposition to the extension of a multiculturalist ethic to medical treatment can be traced to two principles that clinicians themselves have long recognised as ethically indispensable in the justification of medical treatment generally and, more specifically, in regulating the relationship between clinician and patient: the principles of beneficence and non-maleficence. The latter requires that clinicians seek to avoid causing any unnecessary harm to the patient, whereas the former 'asserts an obligation to help others further their important and legitimate interests' (p. 260)[11]. Not surprisingly, clinicians have tended to construe 'harm' and 'interests' in medical terms, as referring primarily, or even exclusively, to the physiological well-being of the patient as determined by the objectively verifiable diagnostic procedures of medicine. On this reading, the relationship between clinician and patient is an unavoidably hierarchical one, to the extent that the clinician's perspective is necessarily accorded priority over that of the patient. The clinician's authority is, to a large extent, grounded in the presumed objectivity of scientific rationality, and this is justified to the extent that the clinician restricts his or her attention to the identification and appropriate treatment of the underlying physiological causes of a given ailment. It follows, however, that clinicians could undermine this authority vested in them should they extend their diagnosis and treatment to include what might be termed medically inappropriate factors, such as the patient's own thoroughly subjective beliefs about the causes of the ailment or about how treatment should proceed. As Helman argues, 'because medicine focuses more on the physical dimensions of illness, factors such as personality, religious belief, culture and socio-economic status of the patient are often considered largely irrelevant in making the diagnosis or prescribing treatment' (p. 81)[4]. Given this, it may seem positively unreasonable to criticise clinicians for claiming to know how a patient's medical interests may best be served. After all, is this not a principal objective of medical training and expertise? Wouldn't one be more justified in criticising a clinician who claimed not to know how a patient's medical interests are best served, than one who did make such a claim? Clearly, if the relationship between clinician and patient was determined entirely by considerations of medical interests, then little, if any, deliberative weight could be accorded to the possible effects that the patient's cultural beliefs and values might have upon diagnosis and treatment. However, there is another ethical principle that has come to exert an increasing influence upon the relationship between clinician and patient: the principle of patient autonomy.

The extension of the principle of respect for patient autonomy contains the potential for significantly altering the relationship between clinician and patient to the extent that it generally restricts the clinician from performing any medical procedures to which the patient has not consented. In accordance with the principle of autonomy, clinicians generally operate under a moral and legal obligation to respect the patients' wishes concerning the forms of medical treatment to which they are to be subjected. One might think of the principle as providing the patient with a veritable right of veto over proposed medical procedures. But, why should the principle of autonomy be accorded such an importance?

A wholly satisfactory answer to this question would entail a lengthy and detailed philosophical discussion, and so far exceed the remit of this chapter.

Suffice it to say that the ideal of personal autonomy has exerted a considerable influence upon the political organisation and regulation of societies such as ours. Indeed, many philosophers have argued that the very legitimacy of the liberal-democratic political system is dependent upon the extent to which such a system facilitates its citizens' exercise of autonomy[9]. The public institutions and services provided by the liberal-democratic state are meant to be regulated in accordance with the principle of respect for autonomy. But what does autonomy consist of? What does it mean to be 'autonomous'?

The essence of autonomy is the notion of self-rule, or self-determination. The philosopher, Isaiah Berlin presents the following definition of autonomy:

> I wish my life and decisions to depend on myself, not on external forces of whatever kind. I wish to be an instrument of my own, not of other men's, acts of will. I wish to be a subject, not an object; to be moved by reasons, by conscious purposes which are my own, not by causes which affect me, as it were, from outside. I wish to be a somebody, not a nobody; a doer – deciding, not being decided for, self-directed and not acted on by external nature or by other men as if I were a thing, or an animal, or a slave incapable of playing a human role, that is, of conceiving goals and policies of my own and realizing them . . . (p. 131)[12].

Berlin's definition of personal autonomy provides a philosophical bedrock upon which subsequent accounts of autonomy have been developed and presented. Specifically, Berlin identifies the possession of a developed self and freedom from external constraints or manipulation as two essential conditions for the exercise of autonomy. However, what is missing from Berlin's account of autonomy is any consideration for the cultural basis and context of human agency and deliberation, or any recognition of the extent to which the actual objects of an individual agent's will are themselves culturally constituted and determined, as philosophers such as Taylor and Raz argue. Indeed, Raz has explicitly argued that the objects of an individual's autonomous deliberation are always culturally constituted phenomena[9]. This is a highly significant point, since what it indicates is the fact that individuals exercise their autonomy precisely through deliberation upon the beliefs and values of the culture(s) with which they identify.

From this standpoint, it follows that the moral obligation to respect a patient's cultural beliefs may be best considered as falling under the aegis of the principle of respect for the patient's autonomy. Thus, what is of principal importance here is not so much the specific character of the cultural beliefs and values in question, but rather the manner in which the patient deliberated upon and arrived at his or her decision. In this way, the obligation to respect a patient's cultural beliefs may be most effectively defended as a constituent part of the principle of respect for autonomy, itself a well-established feature of the ethical regulation of the clinical relationship. Indeed, it certainly seems plausible to conclude that the fundamental beliefs and values of a patient's culture are, on the face of it, a legitimate category of reasons upon which to base a refusal to consent to treatment. A failure or refusal to respect such a decision would clearly amount to a violation of the respect for the autonomy principle, as well as a failure to respect the patient's culture. Does that mean, then, that clinicians must simply step back from their own moral commitments in these circumstances and allow patients to suffer medically preventable deaths or ill-health?

The answer to this question is philosophically complicated and, I must admit, somewhat inconclusive. The respect for the autonomy principle does not require that clinicians unconditionally accept whatever decision a patient arrives at; it is subject to certain, well-established, conditions and limitations. However, it is precisely at this point that the whole question of a patient's cultural affiliation becomes especially problematic, as I shall now explain.

It is clear that if patient autonomy is to consist of more than a validation of the clinician's own decision and will then the implementation of the principle of respect for patient autonomy must allow for the possibility of patients reaching alternative decisions to those recommended by the clinician, even where these decisions take the form of a refusal to consent to essential medical treatment. However, the principle of autonomy does not require clinicians to respect each and every decision made by each and every patient. On the contrary, what it does require is that only the patient's autonomous decisions need be respected. In keeping with the two initial conditions of autonomy identified by Isaiah Berlin referred to above, the crucial questions that follow from this are: was the patient capable of autonomous deliberation; and was this decision free from undue external coercion or manipulation? When combined, these two conditions provide clinicians with a criterion or standard against which to judge whether patients' decisions should be respected.*

---

*Although it should be pointed out that, in proceeding in this way, one is necessarily subsuming the call to respect patients' cultural affiliation within the principle of autonomy. In themselves, reasons based upon the presumed value of culture are thereby denied any 'special' status. This raises a number of very interesting and deeply problematic philosophical questions which, unfortunately, cannot be addressed here.

In so doing, they also provide a means for evaluating the patient's appeal to their cultural affiliation as the principal justificatory ground for their decision.

In respect of the first condition concerning the patient's capacity for the exercise of autonomous choice, the conventional test that has been applied by clinicians is the so-called 'mental competence' test[11]. Typically, this test has been applied in such a manner as to enable clinicians to identify those categories of patients who are deemed to be either permanently or temporarily incapable of exercising autonomous choice, for example, toddlers or those suffering from a serious mental illness. Once classified as incompetent in this respect, clinicians may proceed to administer treatment without requiring the actual consent of the patient concerned provided that doing so is in the interests of the patient. However, the application of this particular test to those refusing treatment on cultural grounds seems very problematic. Indeed, one obvious implication of such a move would be to severely restrict patients' general right of freedom of expression and religious affiliation, given that the exercise of such a right could result in patients being classified as 'mentally incompetent' solely on the basis of the beliefs and values they profess. Not only would this constitute a gross violation of the multiculturalist ethos, it would also involve clinicians engaging in the kind of oppressive practices more commonly associated with the psychiatric services of the former Soviet Union!

In dismissing the 'mental competence test' as valid for the situation being addressed here, one is left with the second condition for determining the extent to which a patient is capable of exercising autonomous choice: the question concerning whether, in making the decision, the patient was free from external coercion or manipulation. In contrast to the first condition, a satisfactory answer to this question will typically require a consideration of the substance of the cultural beliefs and values upon which a patient has based his or her decision. The reason for this may be simply stated. The very nature of some cultural beliefs and values appear to be thoroughly incompatible with the principle of autonomy, in so far as they demand not so much the individual's critical deliberation as unquestioning obedience. Such cultural beliefs and values simply exclude the possibility of an individual legitimately acting in any other way than that prescribed by the fundamental tenets of their culture. Thus, one might identify a category of cultural beliefs and values that exclude the possibility of autonomous deliberation, but to which a patient may appeal in seeking to justify a decision to forego treatment. How should clinicians respond in such instances?

In addressing this question, and in concluding this chapter, I wish to consciously adopt the role of a philosopher who proceeds in the full knowledge that the attempt to identify rationally defensible ethical principles may conflict with the actual practices to which these principles have been or may be applied. As it stands, clinicians are under no strict legal obligation to unconditionally respect the cultural beliefs and values of their patients in cases where such respect will result in patients' medically preventable suffering and death. However, clinicians are under a legal obligation to seek patients' valid consent to proposed medical treatment. This obligation is itself grounded in the principle of respect for autonomy, and the realisation of this principle must allow for the possibility of patients refusing to consent to treatment. However, clinicians are not unconditionally bound to respect patients' decisions.

The crucial test is whether these decisions can be said to be autonomous. Of particular importance in situations where patients cite cultural affiliation as the basis for their decisions is the question of whether they were free from external coercion or manipulation in their deliberations. If this question can be answered in the affirmative then it follows that patients' decisions should be respected in accordance with the autonomy principle. However, one must acknowledge the existence of a category of cultural beliefs and values that prohibit any autonomous deliberation. Although this raises some potentially very problematic issues, it is nevertheless difficult to see, on the basis of the autonomy principle, why clinicians should be compelled to respect patients' decisions to forego essential medical treatment that have been demonstrably based on this category of beliefs and values alone. For this to be ethically acceptable, one would have to either reformulate one's understanding of what constitutes a genuinely 'autonomous' decision or one would have to add another principle to the ethical regulation of medical treatment, one requiring clinicians' to unconditionally respect patients' culturally grounded beliefs and values. Either way, a more ultimately satisfying answer to this particular problem appears to require continuing philosophical exertion.

References

1. Taylor C. Multiculturalism and the Politics of Recognition. Princeton NJ: Princeton University Press, 1992
2. Kukathas C. (ed.) Multicultural Citizens: the philosophy and politics of identity. St. Leonards, NSW: Centre for Independent Studies, 1993
3. Raz J. Multiculturalism. In: Ethics in the Public Domain. J Raz. Oxford: Clarendon Press, 1994
4. Helman CG. Culture, Health and Illness. 4th edn. Oxford: Butterworths, 2000 [esp. Chs 4 & 5]
5. Gillon R. Autonomy and Consent. In: Moral Dilemmas in Modern Medicine. M Lockwood, ed. Oxford: Oxford University Press, 1985
6. Ohnuki-Tierney E. Brain death and organ transplantation: cultural bases of medical technology. Curr Anthropol 1994; 35: 233–54
7. Taylor C. The Politics of Recognition. In: Multiculturalism: a Critical Reader. DT Goldberg, ed. Oxford: Blackwell, 1995
8. Taylor C. Philosophy and the Human Sciences (Philosophical Papers, Vol. 2). Cambridge: Cambridge University Press, 1985
9. Raz J. The Morality of Freedom. Oxford: Oxford University Press, 1986
10. Mendus S. Toleration and the Limits of Liberalism. Basingstoke: Macmillan, 1989
11. Beauchamp T, Childress JF. Principles of Biomedical Ethics. 4th edn. Oxford: Oxford University Press, 1994 [esp. Chs 3, 4 & 5]
12. Berlin I. Four Essays on Liberty. Oxford: Oxford University Press, 1969: 131

Ethical and Legal Issues Affecting the Treatment of Children 6

Nicholas Pace

Introduction

Beauchamp and Childress assert that there are four guiding principles in medical practice: respect for autonomy, beneficence (do good), maleficence (do not harm) and justice (resources have to be distributed fairly)[1]. Of these, the principle of respect for autonomy is becoming increasingly important compared with the other principles, largely due to changes in the value placed in it by society. This does not only apply to adults. As shall be discussed, children are now accorded increased rights, and, hence, they have greater autonomy and a role in the decision-making surrounding their treatment. Knowledge of the ethical and legal issues pertaining to paediatric anaesthesia is important for all practising anaesthetists, particularly in relation to the rights of children and issues of consent and refusal of treatment. Foetal issues, such as their rights, especially in the context of protection and foetal surgery, are an evolving field, and these will not be considered here but are discussed in Chapter 10.

Children's rights

From an ethical viewpoint, moral rights are stringent entitlements yielded by valid moral principles, even if society fails to recognise them[2]. Rules to protect widely agreed values are crucial to every society. Among the modern values so defended is a set of fundamental human rights, central to which are concepts of liberty and self-determination[3]. The benchmark of human rights standards is the *Universal Declaration of Human Rights*, adopted by the United Nations General Assembly in 1948. Human rights' activity attempts to ensure that individuals' rights are not sacrificed in order to benefit society's interests. This is especially important in the conduct of research. The incorporation of the concept of informed consent into research ethical codes is a major consequence of the recognition of human rights. The rights of an individual, however, are not paramount. It may occasionally be necessary to override them in the interests of, for example, public health.

Social change in Europe since the early 1980s has led to children slowly developing human and legal rights of their own, with the consequence that society has obligations towards them. The *United Nations Convention on the Rights of the Child (1976)*[4] stated, in Article 12, that:

> State Parties shall assure to the child who is capable of forming his or her own views the right to express those views freely in all matters affecting the child, the views of the child being given due weight in accordance with the age and maturity of the child.

In 1996, the Parliamentary Assembly of the Council of Europe, in recommendation 1286, strongly urged member states to 'enable the views of children to be heard in all decision-making which affects them'.

Thus, autonomy rights in children are changing, in many countries, from an emphasis on a stated age of consent to interest in individual ability. There is a complex tension, however, between children's autonomy and their right to protection. Children need to be protected from choices that may be harmful to themselves while at the same time respecting their autonomy and right to be involved in decision making. This issue bears heavily on the rights of a child to be involved in decisions regarding his or her health care. How much say in these issues a child may have, especially with regard to refusal of treatment, is controversial.

Consent

All medical interventions require a patient's consent to make them legal. Five conditions are required to make consent acceptable: the patient must be competent, relevant information needs to be disclosed, the information must be understood, the consent must be voluntary and, finally, the patient needs to give authorisation (p. 78)[1]. Of these, the issue of competence is the most important (and controversial) when dealing with children.

Age of competence

A child patient may not be competent to make a decision (and is, therefore, unable to give consent) because he or she is too young. In such situations, a proxy, usually a parent, is entitled to give consent because the law invests such a person that power. The person vested with that power, however, must use it reasonably (p. 222)[5].

In the United Kingdom, a child becomes an adult at the age of 18. A person above this age, provided they are not mentally incapacitated, has the right to make decisions regarding their medical treatment and, indeed, may refuse what is offered, even if the treatment proposed is clearly in that patient's interests. Once a child reaches this age, he or she becomes an adult and is given legal rights to make decisions and may give or refuse consent to whatever medical treatment they wish.

This does not mean that a child who has not yet reached this age (i.e. is under 18) has no legal or ethical rights. Most legal systems throughout the Western world have recognised the concept of the 'mature' or 'emancipated' minor, with the consequent legal capacity to consent to medical treatment. That is, once the child attains a certain level of mental maturity, he or she is entitled to make decisions regarding his or her treatment.

One of the first cases to address this concept was the Canadian case of *Johnston* v. *Wellesley Hospital*[6]. One of the questions raised was whether a minor could consent to treatment. The judge stated that if a minor was old enough to appreciate fully the nature and consequences of the proposed treatment, then he could give effective consent. In another Canadian case (*Catholic Children's Aid Society of Metropolitan Toronto* v. *K*[7]), the trial judge took into account the child's sincerity, maturity and forthrightness and respected the child's wishes rather than those of her legal guardians.

The *Johnston* decision had a direct bearing on the widely known English case of *Gillick* v. *West Norfolk AHA*[8]. Prior to this case the *Family Law Reform Act (1969)*, which had reduced the age of majority from 21 to 18, decreed at section 8, subsection 1, that, once children reached the age of 16, they could consent to any surgical, medical or dental treatment themselves. In other words, adult status was reached at 16 for the purpose of medical treatment and it was, therefore, not necessary to obtain parental consent. The *Gillick* case, however, concerned the validity of consent to contraceptive treatment from a child who was *under* 16, without parental knowledge. The House of Lords ruled that a child under 16 years could give valid consent to medical treatment, without parental consent, provided the child, in the opinion of the doctor, was of sufficient maturity and intelligence to understand the implications of the treatment proposed.

It would, therefore, be up to the individual doctor to decide whether a child under 16 years of age could give valid consent. The basis on which the doctor is to make this decision is, unfortunately, ill defined. It is unlikely this decision will be challenged if made in good faith. However, should it be challenged, then the normal rules of negligence will apply. So, in the UK, if a responsible body of medical opinion agreed that the child was competent to give consent, the action against the doctor should fail. Consequently, in difficult cases, advice from colleagues should be sought. The level of competence required would vary according to the risks involved. In certain situations, such as various heart or neurological operations, it would be highly unlikely that a child could give effective consent. Giesen, an authority on medical malpractice law, believes that when the minor's own future welfare is at stake and the consequences of the procedure might be serious, traumatic or irreversible, physicians should generally seek parental cooperation[9].

Even if the child is deemed not to be of sufficient maturity to consent, it is important that the child participates in the decision-making process, although the final decision would not be theirs. This is in keeping with Article 12 of the *United Nations Convention on the Rights of the Child*. In the UK, however, there is a difference in its interpretation and enforcement. *The Children (Scotland) Act 1995* provides that a parent must, in reaching a decision regarding a child, have regard as is practicable to the views of the child concerned. Furthermore, in section 6, 'a child twelve years of age or more shall be presumed to be of sufficient age and maturity to form a view.' England, together with Wales and Northern Ireland, adopts a more paternalistic approach. In England, in the absence of state intervention, parents have no legal obligation to ascertain or have regard to children's wishes before making decisions, even major ones, which affect the child.

Refusal of treatment

The issue of refusal of treatment by a minor is even more problematic. Following decisions such as *Gillick*[8], it would appear logical that the child has every right to refuse treatment, provided he or she has sufficient maturity and intelligence to understand the implications of refusing the treatment proposed. If one is legally entitled to consent, one must be legally entitled to dissent[10], a situation analogous to the adult situation. Judgement regarding competence would be made by the physician, with advice from colleagues in difficult cases.

However, in the past, the courts and society have consistently failed to accept that a competent child may refuse medical treatment. In many jurisdictions, a minor cannot refuse treatment that, in the opinion of the medical profession or courts, is in his or her best interests. Several test cases have established this precedent[11].

The English case of *Re R*[12] concerned a 15-year-old whose disturbed behaviour required sedation. However, when lucid and competent, she refused her medication. The judges held that the court could override both consent and refusal of treatment if that was considered to be in her best interests. Further, the judges suggested that the parental right to give consent in the face of the child's refusal was retained. This was further considered in the case of *Re W*[13]. This concerned a 16-year-old suffering from anorexia nervosa who was refusing all treatment. Lord Donaldson stated:

> No minor of whatever age has power by refusing consent to treatment to override a consent to treatment by someone who has parental responsibility for the minor . . .

Thus it would appear that a child is mature enough to decide on treatment only if this agrees with what the courts and medical profession wish to do. This is illogical, and these decisions have been widely criticised. For example, it is argued that in some countries a child as young as ten years of age can be held criminally responsible for his or her actions. Yet this same child is not allowed to refuse medical treatment. The child appears to have responsibilities but no rights. The child is said, by refusing treatment, to be acting irrationally. However, the ethical principle of autonomy is about how people are treated and their rights. Acting irrationally does not change their rights. An adult acting irrationally and refusing treatment would have that wish accepted[14]. Children's autonomy should be valued separately from their rationality[15].

However, both cases quoted above were unusual in that they dealt with diseases that could impair reasoning. Indeed, the judges in both cases emphasized the importance of respecting the minor's wishes, and of giving them increasing value with increasing maturity. The concept of the mature minor should, therefore, be breached only in exceptional circumstances (p. 229)[5].

In summary, at least in England, when a child reaches the age of 16, his or her consent will be valid for treatment. This will be overturned if the patient is not competent to consent. Below the age of 16, doctors must assess the particular child's capacity to consent in relation to the proposed intervention. This involves the ability to understand that there is a choice and that choices have consequences. There must be a willingness and ability to make a choice and an ability to understand the nature and purpose of the proposed procedure and the available alternatives, including a proper assessment of the risks and side-effects inherent in these alternatives (p. 286)[16]. The child's decision to withhold consent may be overridden by a parent, legal guardian or the courts.

To confuse the issue, the above does not apply to Scotland. The *Age of Legal Capacity (Scotland) Act 1991* and later the *Children (Scotland) Act 1995* gave young people aged 16 or over the same right to consent or refuse as adults. Furthermore, if a child under the age of 16 is judged competent, the child's consent or refusal should normally be accepted in the same way as an adult's consent or refusal. The child cannot be legally overruled if deemed competent. If there are doubts about the assessment of the child's competence, other opinions should be sought.

It is clear, therefore, that, wherever they are in the UK, practitioners should review each case carefully and in cases of doubt seek legal advice. From a legal point of view, competence is an all-or-nothing issue, that is, one is either competent or incompetent to make a particular decision. The problem revolves around the evaluation of competence and assessing the degree of understanding that the child has in relation to the various aspects of the proposed procedure. Unfortunately, there do not appear to be any guidelines on how this is to be assessed or measured. It is for the doctor to decide whether a minor is competent or not, and it would appear that, if this is challenged, the final arbiter would be whether a responsible body of medical opinion would support the decision taken. Clearly this is very much a grey area in terms of legal obligations, but it appears that the law is taking a back seat and allowing the medical profession to make these decisions. Such a situation, clearly, may change if another controversial case comes before the courts creating a new precedent.

From an ethical viewpoint, the pronouncements of various international bodies have led to an increased awareness of children's rights and autonomy. The *European Convention on Human Rights* will further support the right to self-determination of competent young people. As noted above, minors are not given the full range of rights and choices until they reach the age of majority, usually 18, the age commonly designated as adulthood. There must, therefore, be competing rights, which in turn limit the rights of the child, such as the interests of society and parental rights. The competing interests of the child, parents and the State cannot always be readily reconciled.

Further problems arise when assessing children's rights because such assessments are usually based on autonomy and self-determination. Determining whether a child is competent to take decisions can be complex. Indeed, a child may be deemed competent to consent to treatment but incompetent to refuse that same treatment. This is based on the interests of society in ensuring that young people are not put at risk. Some authors believe, however, that, given adults' tendency to underestimate the abilities of young people, a presumption of competence should be applied[17]. Although considerable progress has been made in recognising children's rights, one can only hope that the admirable principles enshrined in the *UN Convention on the Rights of the Child* will all ultimately be implemented. Perhaps competence should even be specified in statutory form.

The immature minor – who is entitled to give consent?

This is a frequently encountered problem where the child attends for medical or dental treatment accompanied by an adult who is not their parent. The following may give consent on behalf of an incapable child[18]:

- the child's natural mother whether married to the father or not
- the child's natural father whether married or divorced
- an unmarried father who has entered and registered a formal parental responsibilities and parental rights agreement with the mother
- a legal guardian nominated in writing by a parent before the parent's death
- a person holding a court order giving them the right to consent on the child's behalf
- a person who has had delegated to them by a parent/legal guardian the right to consent to medical procedures or treatment of the child
- a person aged 16 years or more who has care and control of the child (e.g. foster carers) except those involved in the setting of school and procedures such as organ donation, non-therapeutic research or treatment (e.g. cosmetic surgery).

Consent by one parent is sufficient, as parents may act independently, unless a court order has been made restricting his or her right to consent (*The Children's Act (1989) s2:7*). As Lord Donaldson (*Re R*[19]) stated:

> . . . if the parents disagree, one consenting and the other refusing, the doctor will be presented with a professional and ethical, but not with a legal problem because, if he has the consent of one authorised person, treatment will not without more constitute a trespass or criminal assault.

Parental refusal of consent

The refusal of medical treatment by parents on grounds of their religious beliefs can be particularly contentious. Article 30 of the *United Nations Convention of the Rights of the Child* suggests that a child belonging to a religious minority shall not be denied the right to practise his or her own religion. On the other hand, article 6 states that every child has a right to life, while article 18 states that the best interests of the child will be the legal guardian's basic concern. Should parental views and rights be overridden by the state?

Parental refusal of treatment is of particular concern to anaesthetists because such examples include refusal of blood transfusions by parents who are Jehovah's Witnesses. Overriding religious convictions is a major step to take in a free society, interfering with the principle that parents should have the freedom to choose the religious and social upbringing of their children (p. 223)[5]. However, as mentioned earlier, the person vested with the power of proxy consent must use it reasonably and, in these cases, the well-being of the child is paramount. Therefore, refusal of life-saving treatment is routinely disregarded, and the law has virtually always allowed the transfusion to be given, overriding the parental objection. If time is available, the approval of a court of law should be sought before such an administration. The Association of Anaesthetists of Great Britain and Ireland (p. 5)[20] suggest that two doctors of consultant status should make an unambiguous, clear and signed entry in the clinical record that blood transfusion is essential, or likely to become so, to save life or prevent serious permanent harm. The parents should be given the opportunity to be properly represented and be kept fully informed of the doctor's intention to apply for a court order (*Re T*[21]). In an emergency, where there is no time to obtain court approval, health professionals should proceed with life-saving treatment, the justification for this being the doctrine of necessity. Treatment should be limited to that which is reasonably necessary.

However, despite the assumption that life-saving treatment can be administered against the wishes of the parents, a few cases have also established the precedent that, in some situations, parents can legally refuse consent to such treatment of their child. In *Couture-Jacquet* v. *Montreal Children's Hospital*[22], a hospital took the mother to court after she had refused chemotherapy for her 3-year-old child who was suffering from cancer. The court upheld the mother's decision because the judges felt there was only a small chance of recovery and also because of the severe side-effects that would result from chemotherapy. Again, it is impossible to set hard and fast rules. Each case should be analysed on its own merits. What is clear is that, if treatment is immediately necessary to preserve life, doctors should proceed with treatment. If treatment is not immediately required then referral to a court of law should be undertaken. Doctors can only act in defiance of parental views in the emergency situation.

Unavailability of parents

As previously discussed, a competent child can give consent for both elective and emergency treatment. If the child is incompetent, however, in the elective situation some form of contact needs to be established with the parents or legal guardian. A telephone contact is acceptable, but it should be witnessed and documented. If contact cannot be established, this should be documented and consideration given as to whether to proceed. This may depend on the seriousness and risks of the proposed procedure. Discuss with senior colleagues is advisable. Good documentation, as always, is essential.

If treatment is required as an emergency it is reasonable to proceed if this is in the best interests of the child and treatment cannot be delayed. Documentation of all discussions should be entered into the case notes.

Under-age mother

This situation, where the parent is herself under 16, is becoming increasingly more common. Assessment of the capacity of the mother to consent on behalf of the child needs to be made. It may also be necessary to include the mother's parents in the consent process, and this should be documented. It is important, however, to be aware that issues of confidentiality may arise.

Non-therapeutic interventions

Assessing benefits and burdens in relation to children's medical treatment can be difficult. Problems are further compounded when assessing the acceptability of non-therapeutic interventions such as organ donation. The limits of parental consent in such situations, when there may be no benefit to the child, are controversial.

Male circumcision   An issue directly applicable to anaesthetists involving religious beliefs is that of male circumcision. In children, this virtually always relies on parental consent. The usual reasons for carrying out the procedure are for ritual, social or cultural purposes. Brazier[23] has commented that male circumcision is a matter of medical debate but that for Jewish and Muslim parents it is an article of faith. Although medical opinion may not necessarily regard it as positively beneficial, it is in no way medically harmful if properly performed as the child suffers only momentary pain. The community as a whole, she claims, regards it as a decision for the infant's parents.

Brazier's comments are open to criticism. Firstly, there is an extensive literature on the harms of circumcision[24]. Secondly, it is not clear from her argument how the operation can be justified legally and ethically. If the principal starting point is that everyone has a right to bodily integrity and, secondly, that proxy consent has to be used reasonably and in the interests of the child, then, clearly, the procedure cannot be justified. It is clear that parental rights are derived from parental duties and exist only so long as they are needed for the protection of the person and property of the child. As Lord Scarman in his judgement in *Gillick*[8] asserted, consent to medical treatment of a child is a clear example of parental responsibility arising from the duty to protect the child. The rights reside with the child and the parents merely act as agents for the child to enforce those rights[25]. Even the argument utilised later when considering non-therapeutic research, which is that it is acceptable so long as it is not *against* the interests of the child, fails because of the harms caused. The UK has not addressed this problem, and it may, therefore, be useful to see how others have considered it. The clearest advice has come from Australia, where the Queensland Law Reform Commission stated:

> Unless there are immediate health benefits to a particular child from circumcision, it is unlikely that the procedure itself could be considered therapeutic . . . The circumcision is invasive, irreversible and major. It involves the removal of an otherwise healthy organ part. It has serious attendant risks . . . On a strict interpretation of the assault provisions of the Queensland Criminal Code, routine circumcision of a male infant could be regarded as a criminal act. Further, consent by parents to the procedure being performed may be invalid in the light of the common law's restrictions on the ability of parents to consent to the non-therapeutic treatment of children[26].

If ever the UK addresses this problem, it might be appropriate to give the Queensland review greater consideration. Finally, those in favour of continuing with this practice need to answer one further question; why can't the procedure wait until the child is old enough to make his or her own decision?

Organ donation   The first kidney transplants were undertaken between identical minors. Couples are now having children for the express purpose of providing genetically compatible sibling donors of, at present, regenerative tissue such as bone marrow. Whether these practices are ethically and legally acceptable is debatable, but it appears that they are likely to increase.

It is unclear whether minors can legally donate tissue in the UK, although the donation of bone marrow between minors is increasingly undertaken. It would appear, from the arguments discussed earlier, that the '*Gillick*' competent minor should be able to consent, subject to the restrictions of that minor understanding the risks and benefits involved. However, whereas this may be acceptable for donating regenerative tissue such as blood, donation of non-regenerative organs such as kidneys involves far greater risks. Similarly, the risks inherent in the surgery to obtain the organs are relevant. It is far riskier to obtain a part of a liver than to obtain bone marrow, despite both being capable of regeneration. Furthermore, Lord Donaldson (*Re W*[13]) stated that:

> It is inconceivable that [the doctor] should proceed in reliance solely upon the consent of an under-age patient, however 'Gillick competent' in the absence of supporting parental consent and equally inconceivable that he should proceed in the absence of the patient's consent. In any event he will need the opinion of other doctors and may well be advised to apply to the court for guidance . . .

The validity of the child's consent would turn on questions such as the seriousness of the intervention, the degree of risk intrinsic in the procedure, the long term implications for the donor and so on. Kennedy and Grubb concluded that it would be a rare child whom the law would find competent to consent to donation of a kidney as against the donation of blood (p. 1761)[27].

The situation regarding incompetent minors is even less clear. The debate hinges around whether parents have the right to consent on behalf of their child to something that will not benefit, and may indeed harm, the child. Once again, the separation into regenerative and non-regenerative tissue helps assess what would be an acceptable risk. What benefits the donor child gains, such as survival of a sibling or parent, will also need to be considered. It is suggested that application to the courts would be needed in most cases in the UK. However, donation of non-regenerative organs from children is generally regarded as being unacceptable, and with regard to partial liver donations most authorities advise that the risks to the paediatric donor of the surgical resection far outweigh the benefits. A number of countries within Europe have specific legislation prohibiting the use of living transplant organ donors while others allow it only after stringent preconditions are satisfied. Mason and McCall Smith believe that no currently practising British transplant surgeon would accept a live child as a solid organ donor (p. 346–7)[5].

Informed consent

The issue of informed consent and information disclosure and understanding is identical to the adult situation, and it is been considered in greater detail elsewhere in this collection (see Chapter 2). Specific written consent forms for anaesthesia are not currently required in the UK. Although consent for anaesthesia is implied when the surgical operation consent form is signed, it is good practice to discuss relevant aspects of the anaesthetic technique to be employed with the child and/or parent and to document this. This is especially important for invasive procedures and for analgesic techniques, such as regional blocks or patient-controlled analgesia. Many centres have written information sheets for parents and children about anaesthesia and analgesic techniques, and this extra information is usually welcomed[28].

Children in research

The aim of research is the generation of new knowledge, but any benefits identified impact on future patients. In the meantime there is potential for the research subject to suffer harm. The incorporation of the concept of informed consent into research ethical codes is a major consequence of the recognition of human rights. Furthermore, whereas in treatment it may be acceptable not to disclose something to a patient (or child) if it is felt that such disclosure may harm the patient, the so-called 'therapeutic privilege', this is not acceptable in research. *Halushka* v. *University of Saskatchewan*[29] established that 'there can be no exceptions to the ordinary requirements of disclosure in the case of research as there may well be in ordinary medical practice.'

It is interesting to note that, whereas in the past the main concern from a human rights point of view was the protection of the research subject from the harms of research, more recently human rights activity has concentrated on campaigning for the majority of the world's populations to be included in some research projects, such as those concerning human immunodeficiency virus

(HIV) infection in Africa. A right can be an entitlement to benefit as well as protecting one's autonomy and liberty.

There are many reasons why it is important that research is undertaken in children. For example, there may be significant differences in pharmacology and physiology that do not allow extrapolation of results from adult research to child therapy. Mere differences, however, do not justify research in children. To be acceptable the research question answered must lead to significant health improvement for children. Indeed, if nothing is to be gained by undertaking research in children it should be undertaken in adults. Also, wherever possible, research should be undertaken in older children.

The issue of undertaking research in children raises many legal and ethical dilemmas. Apart from the fact that they are vulnerable and could be used to further adult interests, questions over what level of maturity is required to consent to a research proposal still arise. Furthermore, harm, pain and distress may arise out of any research, including such simple procedures as taking blood samples. Issues that are also applicable to adult research, such as the use of placebos, study design, research ethics committees and conflicts of interest will not be considered in this chapter.

In the past, research was conveniently divided into 'therapeutic' and 'non-therapeutic', although, in many cases, it was difficult to differentiate the two. Although nowadays this distinction is not routinely used (the preference being a risk : benefit analysis of each component of the research protocol) it can still be very useful when examining the ethical issues concerned. In *therapeutic* research, it is probable (or at least the aim should be) that the research will directly benefit the patient. *Non-therapeutic* research, on the other hand, will not benefit that particular patient, although the results may be very useful in benefiting future patients. It serves as a learning mechanism for the treatment of future patients. In my view, the risk : benefit analysis currently advocated merely emphasises and is part of the therapeutic/non-therapeutic distinction.

Therapeutic research

The question of minors being involved in therapeutic research is not too controversial, and many of the ethical conditions applicable to adult research apply. Consequently, the research doctor has a duty to act in the best interests of the research patient and not to harm them. It is legally wrong for a doctor to withhold information about research therapy for fear that the patient may refuse that therapy, even though the doctor believes it is in the patient's best interest to receive it[30,31].

The 'mature minor' concept discussed earlier, however, confuses the issue slightly. It would appear from the previous discussion that a child who is old enough to understand the risks and implications of involvement in the research project should be ethically and legally entitled to consent. It must be pointed out, however, that this application within the context of research has never been tested in any UK court of law. Furthermore, it is believed a relatively high standard of comprehension by the minor would have to be shown since therapeutic research entails research on a sick child. It could be that the law would not allow such a minor to consent, except when the illness and the research were trivial, because any given minor would lack the necessary maturity to consent. In the case of a minor under the age of 16 years, this would apply with even greater force (p. 1709)[27]. It might also be reasonable for a parent or guardian to override a child's willingness to take part in research that the adult believes to be against the child's interests. There should be no corresponding opportunity for the parent or guardian to override the capable child's refusal (p. 99)[32].

Concerning 'immature minors', parents must give voluntary consent, fully understanding the risks and benefits of the research proposed. The limits of this authority to consent must reflect the risk : benefit analysis of participation in the trial. After assessing this risk : benefit ratio, they must believe that it is in the minor's best interest to be involved in that study. They can then consent on behalf of the minor.

Non-therapeutic research

The question of non-therapeutic research (i.e. research that will not directly treat the patient, although the results may benefit other patients), is much more controversial. Two issues arise: can a proxy lawfully volunteer a minor into a non-therapeutic trial and, if so, are there limits to the risks to be allowed?

Parents are given legal authority to consent on behalf of their children. However, this power cannot be used to harm the child. By definition, a child does not gain directly by being involved in non-therapeutic research and, indeed, may be harmed. This implies that parents cannot consent to their children being involved in non-therapeutic research. In the UK, in 1964, the Medical Research Council[33] stated that:

... in the strict view of the law, parents and guardians of minors cannot give consent on their behalf to any procedures which are of no particular benefit to them and which might carry some risk of harm.

Thus it has been suggested that it appears to be extremely doubtful whether valid consent in non-therapeutic research can be given by proxies on behalf of their child because it cannot be in the child's best interests[9].

There are counter arguments to all of this. Firstly, there are no specific legal rules or rulings on which to base this view[34]. In the UK, there are no statutes or court decisions to help doctors involved in paediatric research (p. 372)[5]. From an ethical point of view, it is claimed that, in everyday life, society allows parents a certain amount of discretion when subjecting their offspring to risks[35]. Therefore, the 'reasonable parent test', employed by Lord Reid in S v. S[36], could be used to support the view that reasonable parents may be allowed to subject their children to certain types of non-therapeutic research, especially where the risk : benefit ratio is highly in favour of large potential benefits to others. Extrapolating from this, many believe that the test should be whether the parents are 'clearly not acting against the best interests of the child'[5].

The extreme arguments advocating no research at all or justifying it as a duty to society are not acceptable. The middle of the road attitude of balancing the risks to the child with the many advantages to society as a whole should prevail. If risks are significant, research should not be allowed, because this would clearly be acting against the best interests of the child.

The British Paediatric Association has stated that it would be unethical to submit a child to more than minimal risk when the procedure offers no benefit to them[37]. They define minimal as procedures such as questioning, observing and measuring children, provided that procedures are carried out in a sensitive way and that consent has been given. It should be noted that, in all cases, when parental consent is obtained, the agreement of school-age children should also be obtained by the researchers. Procedures with minimal risk include collecting a single urine sample (but not by aspiration), or using blood from a sample that has been taken as part of treatment. It is to be noted that taking a sample of blood from a vein, purely for research purposes, was considered to be low risk rather than a minimal risk. However, arguably the use of local anaesthetic creams now allows blood to be drawn with minimal discomfort and, hence, minimal risk.

The Institute of Medical Ethics has defined minimal as a risk of death lower than $1:1\,000\,000$, a risk of major complications less than $1:100\,000$ and a risk of minor complications of less than $1:1000$ (p. 8)[38]. Thus, it could be argued that this level of risk is no greater than those encountered in everyday life.

With regard to mature minors, it could again be argued that they should be allowed to decide for themselves in the same way that adults are allowed, with one limitation, that the greater the risk to the child, the older he or she must be before a doctor decides he or she is 'mature'. Once again, this has never been tested in a UK court of law. An even higher standard of comprehension by the minor would have to be shown than applies to therapeutic research.

Parental presence in the anaesthetic and resuscitation rooms

The issue of parental presence in the anaesthetic room and resuscitation room has also been raised recently. Some argue that a parent has a right to be present during the resuscitation of his or her child, if they so wish. Others argue that the experience of seeing one's child in such a desperate situation (particularly during resuscitation) is likely to cause serious emotional trauma, immediately and in later life. Whenever possible, the wishes of the parents should be respected, however, the anaesthesiologist or resuscitation coordinator should have the final veto. This situation has, as yet, not been challenged in the courts.

Paediatric intensive care

Decision making in the paediatric intensive care unit is more complex than in the adult unit, involving parents or guardians acting as advocates for the child. It is impossible to give a full account of the ethics regarding controversies about withholding and withdrawing treatment in children in the limited space available. The Royal College of Paediatrics and Child Health in the UK, however, has issued guidelines on how to approach such decisions[39] and a summary is provided below.

There are five situations where withholding or withdrawing curative medical treatment might be considered:

1. *The brain dead child.* The criteria for establishing brainstem death are, in principle, the same in children over 2 months of age as in adults. It is rarely possible to diagnose brainstem death in infants less than 2 months of age, and for babies less than 37 weeks post-conceptual age the concept of brainstem death is probably inappropriate. Where criteria of brainstem death are agreed by two practitioners in the usual way it may still be technically feasible to provide basic cardio-respiratory support by means of ventilation and intensive care. It is agreed within the profession that treatment in such circumstances is futile and withdrawal of current medical treatment is appropriate. It is interesting to note that brainstem death criteria have no legal basis. The concept is accepted by the medical profession, and, in turn, the law accepts the profession's view that the patient is legally dead.

2. *The permanent vegetative state.* The child who develops a permanent vegetative state following insults, such as trauma or hypoxia, is reliant on others for all care and does not react to or relate with the outside world. It may be appropriate both to withdraw current therapy and to withhold further curative treatment. It must be noted that, in these cases, the law in most countries wishes to be involved in the decision-making process of withdrawing treatment.

3. *The 'no chance' situation.* The child has such severe disease that life-sustaining treatment simply delays death without any significant alleviation of suffering. Medical treatment in this situation may, therefore, be deemed inappropriate.

4. *The 'no purpose' situation.* Although the patient may be able to survive with treatment, the degree of physical or mental impairment will be so great that it is unreasonable to expect them to bear it. The child in this situation will never be capable of taking part in decisions regarding treatment or its withdrawal.

5. *The 'unbearable' situation.* The child and/or family feel that in the face of progressive and irreversible illness *further* treatment is more than can be borne. They wish to have a particular treatment withdrawn or to refuse further treatment irrespective of the medical opinion on its potential benefit. Oncology patients who are offered further aggressive treatment might be included in this category. The assessment of competence of the child referred to above would once again apply.

In situations that do not fit with these five categories, or where there is dissent or uncertainty about the degree of future impairment, the child's life should always be safeguarded by *all* in the health-care team in the best possible way. Clearly, the recognition that the management of any patient is undertaken, not by medical staff acting on their own, but by a health-care team that also involves nurses, physiotherapists, social workers, etc., means that a team approach that fully integrates the wishes of the child and family is essential.

Decisions must never be rushed, and they must always be made by the team with all evidence available. In emergencies, it is often doctors in training who are called to resuscitate. Rigid rules, even for conditions that seem hopeless, should be avoided; life-sustaining treatment should be administered and continued until a senior and more experienced doctor arrives.

The decision to withhold or withdraw curative therapy should always be followed by consideration of the child's palliative or terminal care needs. These may be related to symptom alleviation (e.g. analgesia or anticonvulsant therapy) or to dignified and comforting nursing care.

Conclusion

Ethical and legal issues pertaining to paediatrics are complicated by the special vulnerability of the subjects. The definition of competence, which in turn influences the law, creates uncertainty. Religious beliefs and social demands merely serve to confuse further, and it remains very difficult to give precise answers to many of the questions that paediatric anaesthetists would like answered. Ethical beliefs change with time and what is currently thought ethically acceptable was not necessarily so a few years ago, and vice-versa. The whole subject of genetics clearly illustrates this. The law tends to change very slowly, and it takes time to catch up with current ethical thinking. The answers to many of the issues raised are, therefore, constantly changing.

References

1. Beauchamp TL, Childress JF. Principles of Biomedical Ethics. Oxford University Press, 1989
2. Held V. Rights and Goods: Justifying Social Action. New York: Free Press, 1984
3. Sommerville A. Informed consent and human rights in medical research. In: Informed Consent in Medical Research. L Doyal, JS Tobias, eds. London: BMA books, 2000: 249–56
4. United Nations Convention on the Rights of the Child (20. xi. 1989; TS44; Cm 1976)
5. Mason JK, McCall Smith RA. Law and Medical Ethics. 4th edn. London: Butterworths, 1994
6. *Johnston* v. *Wellesley Hospital* [1971] 2 OR103, (1970) 17DLR3d 139 (Ont HC)
7. *Catholic Children's Aid Society of Metropolitan Toronto* v. *K* [1985] 47 RFL2d 361 (Ont Dist Ct)
8. *Gillick* v. *West Norfolk AHA* [1984] 1 All ER 365, (1985) 3 ALL ER 402, HL
9. Giesen D. International Medical Malpractice Law. Tubigen: JCB Mohr, 1988
10. Hoggett B. Parents, children and medical treatment: the legal issues. In: Rights and wrongs in medicine. P Byrne, ed. London: King's Fund, 1986
11. Douglas G. The Retreat from Gillick Modern Law Review. 1992; 55: 569–73
12. *Re R* (a minor) (wardship : medical treatment) [1992] Fam11, (1992) 7 BMLR 147, CA
13. *Re W* (a minor) (medical treatment) [1992] 4 All ER 627, (1992) 9 BMLR 22
14. Dickerson D. Children's informed consent to treatment: is the law an ass? J Med Ethics 1994; 20: 205–6, 222
15. Eekelaar J. The interests of the child and the child's wishes. In: The Best Interests of the Child. P Alson, ed. Oxford: Oxford University Press, 1994
16. Montgomery J. Health Care Law. Oxford: Oxford University Press, 1997

17. Alderson P, Montgomery J. Health Care Choices: Making Decisions with Children. London: Institute for Public Policy Research, 1996
18. Edgar J, Morton, NS, Pace NA. Review of Ethics in Paediatric Anaesthesia: Consent Issues. Paediat Anaesth 2001; 11: 3, 355–9
19. *Re R* [1991] 4 All ER 184
20. Association of Anaesthetists of Great Britain and Ireland. Management of Anaesthesia for Jehovah's Witnesses. AAGBI, 1999
21. *Re T.* All ER 1992; 4: 647–70
22. *Couture-Jacquet* v. *Montreal Children's Hospital* (1986) 28 DLR4th 22 (Que CA)
23. Brazier M. Medicine, Patients and the Law. Penguin, 1992
24. Williams N, Kapila L. Complications of circumcision. Br J Surg 1993; 80: 1231–6
25. Dwyer JG. Parents' religion and children's welfare: debunking the doctrine of parents' rights. California Law Rev 1994; 82:1371
26. Circumcision of Male Infants Research Paper. (Chairman: Williams GN). Brisbane: Queensland Law reform Commission, 1993: 39
27. Kennedy I, Grubb A. Medical Law. 3rd edn. London: Butterworths, 2000
28. Association of Anaesthetists of Great Britain and Ireland. Consent for Anaesthesia. London: AAGBI, 1999
29. *Halushka* v. *University of Saskatchewan* (1965) 53 DLR (2d) 436
30. BGH (1984) 7 Feb 1984 (VI ZR 174/82) BGHZ 90, 103 (107–8, 111)
31. Pace N. Medicolegal and ethical issues. In: Pediatric Anesthesia. B Bissonnette, B Dalens, eds. New York: McGraw-Hill, 2002: 1479–85
32. Evans D, Evans M. A Decent Proposal: Ethical Review of Clinical Research. Chichester: J Wiley and Sons, 1996
33. Medical Research Council. Responsibilities in investigations on human subjects. In: Reporting of the Medical Research Council for the year 1962–3. London: HMSO, 1964
34. Dworkin G. Legality of consent to nontherapeutic medical research on infants and young children. Arch Dis Childhood 1978; 53: 443–6
35. Skegg PDG. Law, Ethics and Medicine. Clarendon Press, 1984
36. *S* v. *S* (1970) 3 All ER 107, HL
37. British Paediatric Association. Guidelines for the Ethical Conduct of Medical Research Involving Children. London: BPA, 1992
38. Institute of Medical Ethics. Medical Research with Children: Ethics, Law and Practice. Bull Med Ethics 1996; 14: 8
39. Royal College of Paediatrics and Child Health. Withholding or withdrawing life saving treatment in children: A framework for practice. Summarised in: Bull Med Ethics 1997; 131: 4–5

Clinical Research　　　　7

Michael Harmer

Introduction

Research is, and always has been, an essential part of medical practice and progress. Vital discoveries made over the centuries have certainly changed our lives and our expectations, but not all research has been undertaken in an ethical manner (certainly not by today's standards). Some modern medical knowledge results from research undertaken on unconsenting, often vulnerable, groups of patients and non-patients. We cannot rectify past events but we can regret them, and certainly we all (researchers, doctors, other health-care professions and public alike) have a duty to ensure that there is no repetition.

The General Medical Council (GMC) makes the ethical duties of clinical researchers clear:

> Doctors involved in research have an ethical duty to show respect for human
> life and respect peoples' autonomy. Partnership between participants and the
> health care team is essential to good research practice and such partnerships
> are based on trust. You must respect patients' and volunteers' rights to make
> decisions about their involvement in research. It is essential to listen to and
> share information with them, respect their privacy and dignity, and treat
> them politely and considerately at all times. (p. 2)[1]

In the UK, studies involving humans must be approved by Local Research Ethics Committees (LRECs) or, when more than five centres are involved, Multicentre Research Ethics Committees (MRECs). The LREC/MREC system (or overseas equivalent) is designed to protect patients, investigators and institutions as well as promote trust and public confidence in the scientific process (see Chapter 8).

The scope of clinical research

It is important to understand what the term 'clinical research' means. Whilst laboratory investigations involving *in vitro* or animal studies are of vital importance to the discovery and development of drugs and techniques, they will not be included in the ethical considerations of clinical research. That is not to say that researchers do not have clear responsibilities for ensuring the appropriate level of care in animal studies. Clinical research does, however, include activity outside simple pharmaceutical studies undertaken on consenting adult patients. It includes any investigation into the causes, treatment or prevention of ill health and disease in humans, whether that investigation involves people, their tissues or organs, or data (an area of increasing importance as more and more clinical data are available about individuals). It also includes toxicology studies, clinical trials, genetic studies, epidemiological research including analyses of medical records, and other collections and analyses of data about health and illness, whether anonymised or not.

Although this is a distinction abandoned in the most recent *Declaration of Helsinki*[2], clinical research can be divided into two major categories: therapeutic (where the research may be of potential benefit to participants) and non-therapeutic (where there is no predicted benefit to participants). A distinction is also drawn between clinical research and audit and, accordingly, audit projects are not subject to stringent research ethics scrutiny. The ethical issues related to these latter distinctions are discussed below.

Therapeutic research

Research where there is potential, immediate benefit to the participant is a major part of clinical research activity, for example, comparing a new agent believed to have improved efficacy with the standard available therapy. The comparator can range, however, from placebo (no effective treatment) to the 'gold standard' (the currently accepted *optimal* treatment). Whilst most studies in this category are concerned primarily with efficacy, safety is also important, and any research must ensure that the foreseeable risks associated with the medication, or technique, will not outweigh the potential benefits to the participant. As the GMC clearly states: 'the development of treatments and furthering of knowledge should never take precedence over the patients' best interests' (p. 4)[1].

There are certain prerequisites that have to be fulfilled before undertaking clinical research. Before a new drug is studied to confirm its effectiveness in a particular condition, evidence must be provided of the drug's activity in that condition. This evidence generally comes from initial animal studies (which should also have excluded major unacceptable effects) and studies using healthy volunteers to confirm the safety of the drug and to obtain some estimate of its activity. Studies using healthy volunteers are classed as non-therapeutic research and are discussed below.

The trial design itself may raise ethical issues: for instance, in the choice of comparator used to judge a new agent or technique. Of particular concern is the use of placebo comparators. Using a placebo comparator in the development of a new mouthwash to counter dental plaque development may be relatively uncontroversial. Where the drug is a new analgesic and the condition under investigation is severe post-operative pain, there is more controversy because of the potential harm to the patient.

Placebo comparators

The use of a placebo comparator in a study involving severe post-operative pain is unethical unless its design also ensures effective analgesia for the patient. For instance, the efficacy of the new drug can be assessed not in terms of the patient's experience of pain but by the difference in subsequent analgesic consumption by the patient. This, in turn, can be measured by the time it takes for the patient to request readily-available analgesia, or by actually recording analgesic consumption over a period of time (which is easily facilitated by patient-controlled analgesia systems that ensure that the patient has free access to as much analgesic drug as they feel appropriate for the pain experienced). Such 'analgesic-sparing' studies have become an accepted methodology in the investigation of new analgesics where a placebo arm is required. Similar study design is recommended when two active drugs are compared, particularly if there is some evidence to suggest that the potency of one drug is superior to the other.

Although it is now common practice to ensure that trail designs take account of the harm of unattended pain, it has taken longer for other kinds of discomfort to be recognised as harmful side-effects of research. Over the past decade there has been a heightened awareness of the unpleasant and deleterious effects of post-operative nausea and vomiting, yet placebo-comparator studies have, until recently, been an accepted methodology for the investigation of newer agents[3,4]. Given that nausea and vomiting may be just as unpleasant as pain, there must be major ethical concerns over such studies, and more recent investigations have used study designs similar to those for analgesic studies where, for placebo-controlled studies, there is ready access to effective anti-emetic therapy for the patient during the study period, and efficacy is judged by anti-emetic consumption.

Active comparators

Arguably, if the efficacy and safety of a new drug is to be fully established it has to be compared to a 'gold standard'. In some areas of clinical practice this may not be difficult as there is a clear, accepted current best practice. However, in some areas, there is no obvious or single 'gold standard' and care must be taken to ensure that the established comparator is the most efficacious drug in the setting of the study. An example might be the comparison of a new anti-emetic agent with an established drug for the prevention of opioid-induced nausea and vomiting. There are many anti-emetic drugs available but to choose an agent that has its greatest effectiveness against motion sickness but limited effect against opioids, such as hyoscine, is hardly a true comparison. The temptation to design a study to ensure superiority of a new drug over an existing agent is obvious, but to recruit subjects to a study where the result, by design, is a foregone conclusion is unethical.

Expectations

A further ethical issue in therapeutic research is the raising of a subject's expectations. This is most likely to occur at the time of obtaining consent, when it is very easy to imply, be it unintentionally, that the research involves a 'new, improved' drug whereas the purpose of the study is to establish its efficacy. It is vitally important when obtaining consent to avoid any statement that may

95

influence expectation. The matter of obtaining consent for research projects is dealt with in greater detail below.

Non-therapeutic research

In contrast to the situation in therapeutic research, where the researcher should try to ensure that any risks are less than the potential benefits to the subjects, in non-therapeutic studies where there is no immediate benefit to the participant, the researcher must keep the foreseeable risks to an absolute minimum. In addition, foreseeable risks must be far outweighed by the future potential benefits from the development of treatments and furthering of knowledge.

Recruitment of volunteers

Non-therapeutic studies of new agents are often undertaken prior to full investigation in the clinical setting, and they usually concentrate on side-effect profiles of the drug and safety rather than efficacy. Such studies are often undertaken on volunteers, and this can raise significant ethical issues. While it should be obvious that the ethical dilemma of risk against potential benefit must be considered, the matter of inducement to participate is just as important. Volunteers in non-therapeutic studies may be recruited from one's colleagues, from a student body, from a patient cohort or following advertisement to the general public. The only appropriate volunteers are those who are participating in the full understanding of the importance of the study and for humanitarian reasons. Inappropriate, and unacceptable, subjects are those for whom the inducement for participation will influence their sense of responsibility for themselves. The payment of a large sum of money is, therefore, unacceptable – an example might be the offer of several thousand pounds to have one's heart rendered asystolic and then receive an experimental drug whose purpose is to reverse the effect. Payment of reasonable expenses to cover travelling costs, inconvenience and, possibly, loss of earnings is acceptable. Experimentation on groups such as prisoners with the incentive of reduction in sentence duration is considered by most people to be unethical. It is difficult to justify the recruit of incompetent people for non-therapeutic research.

Clinical non-therapeutic research

Some types of non-therapeutic research involve an extended period of unnecessary treatment or additional instrumentation for the participant so that a phenomenon unrelated to an existing condition can be investigated. An example might be the study of cerebral oxygenation during different types of heart surgery where additional external and intravascular monitors, not necessary for the operative procedure or the anaesthetic, are used to investigate the changes occurring during the different phases of the anaesthetic and surgery. For the participant, there is clearly no immediate benefit and a small additional risk from the invasive monitoring. The potential benefit for the future care of patients undergoing this type of surgery may, however, be significant. Before granting approval, research ethics committees generally require assurance about the safety of invasive techniques employed in such studies, and also confirmation that a less invasive technique would not be feasible.

Audit versus research

Audit is an integral part of normal clinical practice, and evidence of participation in such activity is sought at all levels of seniority. The principle of the classic 'audit cycle' is simple: it is a local procedure where a particular aspect of care is assessed, compared with an established example of 'best practice', any necessary changes made and the resultant service re-examined. This process is local by design to ensure quality of health-care provision and, as such, it does not need approval from a research ethics committee. Unfortunately, some people try to circumvent the research ethics committee and its complicated application forms by declaring a research project to be audit.

There are basically two situations where an investigation is reported as audit when it is, in fact, research. In the first, the researchers are clearly undertaking research because they are not looking at current practice and comparing it with a standard but are introducing a new technique or drug and comparing it with an accepted standard, for example, the evaluation of a new piece of anaesthetic equipment that, whilst freely available, is not the equipment normally used at that hospital. There is normally no deliberate intention on the part of the researcher to deceive and, in some circumstances, researchers are advised by the research ethics committee that its approval is not necessary for such projects. Even allowing for that degree of variability in interpretation, it would seem prudent to obtain a separate consent from participating patients.

The second instance is where a perfectly reasonable local audit project has been undertaken and the results have highlighted something that the investigators feel is worthy of publication and further dissemination. The difficulty here is that the data was gathered for local use (audit), but to publish even anonymised data, research ethics committee approval is required, precisely as it is for research involving previous medical records. Consent is also necessary (see below).

Scientific journal editors are increasingly sensitive to these situations, and they are more likely to reject studies that started as audits (but were then submitted for publication) or were always research masquerading as audit. Prior to undertaking an audit project, individuals should consider whether the project is, in fact, research or whether there might be findings that warrant publication. Under these circumstances, it is prudent to seek advice from the LREC and, irrespective of the advice given, obtain separate consent from participating patients.

Consent

Consent for participation in a research study is similar to consent for medical treatment (see Chapter 2). The main difference is that there is a greater emphasis on information: patients or volunteers must have sufficient, appropriate information in order to decide whether or not to participate in the study.

Types of consent

Consent can be implied or explicit, verbal or written. Sometimes implied consent is sufficient, such as when an injection is given to administer an analgesic. Specific consent for that procedure is not obtained because it is assumed that the patient in making a request for analgesia was aware of the method of delivery. However, for anything more major, and certainly for any operative procedure, explicit consent is required. In order to obtain explicit consent, it is important to ensure that the specific procedure is explained and agreed.

Exactly the same principle applies to consent in research. The subjects must be informed that they are being invited to take part in research, of exactly what will happen and what their involvement will be. They must be given sufficient detail to allow an informed decision. Any foreseeable risks must be identified and, as far as possible, quantified in the information provided. Equally, any possible benefits of the research must be put in context and not exaggerated to influence recruitment. A copy of the information should be given to the patient for their retention. The information must be provided in a format and language that is understandable to the participant and should avoid any unnecessary use of medical terminology.

Verbal and oral consent are equally valid in law but, for the purpose of research, the written format is preferred so that both participant and researcher have a clear written record of what was agreed. The consent document should give details of the information provided and should confirm that the subject has received sufficient information and had sufficient time in which to make a decision. Participants have the right to withdraw from the study at any time without giving a reason, and they should be reassured that their care will not be influenced by a decision to withdraw. It is good practice to have any consent document countersigned by an independent witness not involved in the study design or conduct. That person could be related to the participant or could be a member of the staff not involved in the project.

It is generally inappropriate for consent to be sought immediately prior to the start of the study. In the past, patients have been approached just prior to the induction of anaesthesia, hardly a time when a patient is in an appropriate frame of mind to consider the additional information and make an informed decision. There is also a reasonable chance that the patient will have received some form of sedative pre-medication that may influence his or her ability to make a competent decision. Best practice suggests that 24 hours should be allowed between approaching the patient to seek participation and the start of the study. This allows patients both to give the matter personal consideration and also to seek advice from friends or relatives. For surgical patients, this used to be a relatively easy guideline to accommodate as most patients were admitted to hospital on the day before surgery, however, now patients for major surgery are often admitted on the day of surgery and, accordingly, some mechanism must be developed to ensure that patients have adequate time in which to consider participation. It may be that the project can be broached with them several weeks or months before if they are attending a pre-admission clinic, or, for obstetric studies, during a visit to the antenatal clinic. It is important though to ensure that any agreement to participation in a study made at that time is confirmed at the time of admission to hospital.

Clinical research involving organs, tissues or body fluids

Some types of clinical research involve samples from organs, tissues or body fluids. The most commonly used body fluid is blood, and it is taken to identify the amount of a specific substance within the sample, be that physiological or pharmacological. If samples are to be taken as part of a study, the reason must be made clear to the participant during the consent process. Once a result is available the remainder of the sample is usually destroyed. However, in some cases, and more particularly with organ or tissue samples, the specimen may be retained for a period of time. If, at a later date, a researcher wishes to conduct another study on these samples, additional consent must be obtained from the subject. For example, it is unacceptable for blood samples taken for routine pre-study haematological screening to be used subsequently to investigate the prevalence of a condition, perhaps human immunodeficiency virus (HIV), in this particular population. Clearly, if samples have been kept for some time, there may be logistical problems locating the 'owner'.

Conflicts of Interest

Personal conflicts

It is very easy for researchers to become so involved in their work that they fail to realise that a conflict of interest is developing. These may arise due to pure enthusiasm, perhaps in a situation where the researcher has developed a new technique or manoeuvre and wishes to show that it is an improvement over the existing method. Enthusiasm is understandable, but it can influence the conduct of a study and lead to a biased outcome. It is preferable for any interim analysis to be conducted by independent investigators. It is not uncommon when a new piece of equipment is developed for initial reports to present it in a very favourable light. Later independent studies, however, may be far less favourable, and probably more accurate, in their assessment. Personal enthusiasm and expertise are not unethical per se, but attempts to manipulate recruitment or amend results certainly are.

Financial conflicts

Pharmaceutical companies undertake a great deal of clinical research, and significant amounts of money are paid to institutions for such work. It is essential that every effort is made to ensure that financial gain does not influence the course of an otherwise properly designed and conducted study. Financial arrangements should never be for an individual's benefit but should be targeted at supporting research within an appropriate grouping. It is unethical to attempt to cajole subjects into participation for the researcher's financial gain. It is equally important that any financial support is declared when consent is sought from the patient or volunteer. Finally, the actual sum obtained for such studies should be commensurate with the time, effort and cost of the investigation.

Confidentiality

It is a fundamental principle of clinical research, as with clinical medicine, that any patient or volunteer participating in a project will have their privacy and autonomy respected. Ideally, all data from clinical research should be anonymised unless specific personal data are essential. In such a case, specific consent for any disclosure must be obtained from the participants. It is essential that access to any patient-related data is limited to those directly involved in the study and is not available to others without specific consent from the subject. In virtually all respects, clinical research data must be handled in exactly the same way as other types of personal data and must fulfil the requirements of the *Data Protection Act (1998)* (see Chapter 4).

Recording research results

Researchers have a duty to maintain complete and accurate records, which should include everything involved in the project from the original protocol to the data collection tools used. Such information should be retained in a secure place, and it may be required for future independent audit. In some studies, particularly those sponsored by pharmaceutical companies, records should be preserved for an extended period of up to 15 years and in a manner that preserves confidentiality.

Researchers also have a responsibility to report any adverse events as soon as possible to all involved in the research. This should include any funding bodies, the research ethics committee and the appropriate licensing authority (the Medicines Control Agency for drugs and the Medical Devices Agency for equipment).

Once the project is completed and any randomising code has been broken, the researcher has a duty to inform any participant of the outcome of the research or make the information publicly available.

Use of existing records in research

Retrospective research projects often involved a 'trawl' through appropriate patients' clinical records and, until recently, such studies have not required research ethics committee approval. Now approval is required for all studies involving patient records, with only very few exceptions (some epidemiological studies, and health surveillance studies where notifiable diseases are involved). Exceptional circumstances aside, approval will only be granted if the research undertakes to obtain the patients' consent. This is because records made for one purpose, for example the provision of care, cannot be used for another purpose without undermining the original consent, hence the need for a revised consent. Where is it impossible or ethically undesirable to gain consent, approval usually requires the data to be anonymised before it is used.

Research in vulnerable patients

For the purposes of considering research, 'vulnerable' means anyone who lacks the capacity to consent; for example, young children, mentally disabled people and unconscious patients. Although such patients cannot volunteer for research, it is arguable that they are as entitled to derive medical benefit from research as competent patients. As they are unable to consent to the associated risks, however, in all but exceptional circumstances they should not be included in non-therapeutic research. In order to protect their interests, any therapeutic research should have as its control the standard available therapy – as a minimum. Moreover, because they are unable to make their own decision about the balance of risks and benefits in research, no research should be undertaken on incompetent patients that could be undertaken on competent patients. Unless this is impossible, an additional prerequisite for approval is that similar research has already been undertaken on competent patients.

The particular problems associated with gaining consent from, or for, children are discussed in Chapter 6, and, as stated in that chapter, children cannot consent, and consent cannot be given on their behalf, for research that contains more than an minimal risk of harm, or is against their interests.

There is no legal proxy for adults who lack the competence to consent for themselves. The same principle that governs clinical practice governs recruitment to research trials, namely, that in the opinion of the treating clinician the intervention must be in the interests of the patient. Provided that only minimal risk is involved, incompetent adults may be recruited if it is not *against* their interests to participate. It is common practice for researchers to obtain the assent of someone close to the patient who is in a good position to represent their best interests. This assent carries no legal weight or protection, and it should only be viewed as an additional precaution in the process of determining best interests (see also Chapter 8).

Unconscious adult patients are a sub-group of incompetent adults but raise different ethical issues when there is the possibility that they may regain the capacity to consent. In addition, patients receiving intensive or emergency therapy may have cardiovascular instability and organ dysfunction that pose problems for study design, and may be life-threatening for the patients themselves. Like other incompetent adults, unconscious patients are unable to consent in advance of being involved in a trial. Ideally, one would wait until they regained capacity but this would inevitably exclude them from any trial of therapy for conditions that are critical and, by implication, all research of this kind. Like research on other vulnerable groups, a compromise has to be reached that both protects the patient and enables potentially beneficial research to proceed. The outstanding difficulty that remains is what to do when the patient regains consciousness. For instance, it would be good practice to inform patients that they have been involved in the trial and try to gain their retrospective approval. Presumably, however, a patient could refuse and effectively withdraw from the trial. But discarding information from such patients introduces an element of bias that might undermine the trial design. This is an issue that is in need of more consideration than there is space for here.

Obstetrics

Pregnancy per se is not sufficient for a woman to be considered a vulnerable research subject, but, arguably, the foetus itself is a vulnerable subject and the potential risks of research to the foetus have special resonance post-thalidomide. The difficulties of research on pregnant women are: first, that the risks involved might affect not one but two individuals; and second, that the risks to the foetus might be extremely difficult to quantify.

In considering research relevant to anaesthetic practice, projects rarely involve women in the first or second trimesters of pregnancy: indeed, because this is a vital time for foetal development, very little research at all is carried out during this time. The vast majority of anaesthetic-related research will be undertaken in one of three situations: during labour, intra-operatively or post-operatively. The situation for research in an elective surgical setting (such as elective Caesarean section) is relatively simple as ample time is available for the researcher and woman (and relatives) to discuss the study and for proper consent to be obtained. The woman's main concern in any study is likely to be any potential effect upon the foetus, and particular emphasis must be placed on that aspect in providing information to the mother. Given these considerations, research in the immediate pre-operative and operative settings is relatively straightforward, and it should not raise major ethical concerns.

Most drugs are transferred from the mother to baby through breast milk, and seemingly harmless substances given to mothers may have enhanced or adverse effects once they find their way into the newborn, who is unable to metabolise drugs to the same extent as the mother. Accordingly, in the post-operative period, research (usually involving provision of pain relief) must still give consideration to the possible effects upon the child if the mother is breast-feeding. With this aspect considered, research should not be an ethical problem in the elective setting for there is adequate time available to obtain informed consent.

In terms of consent, the most problematic period for research in obstetrics is during labour, and for anaesthetic practice this usually means the provision of pain relief. As with other analgesic studies, there must be active comparators or a readily identifiable rescue analgesic regimen available. Consent for participation in a study of analgesia in labour cannot be obtained during labour for three reasons. First, the mother will not have had adequate time to consider the proposed study nor to consult with friends and relatives. Second, she may have already received drugs, such as pethidine, that could alter her ability to understand fully the implications of the study. Third, at a time when the mother is in pain, a study presented to her that will relieve pain can be seen as an inappropriate inducement to recruitment. For these reasons, studies in labour have posed problems to researchers and ethics committees alike. There is no universally accepted methodology for such studies, but some maternity consumer groups have produced guidelines for research that make the conduct of studies even more difficult[5]. Standard practice, however, is to obtain a woman's consent to research during labour at the time of a routine antenatal clinic. This gives her time to consider whether to participate, and at a time where her capacity is unimpaired. All the previously discussed aspects of information giving and consent would also apply, including the right to withdraw at any time before or during labour. When a woman who has previously expressed an interest in participation in research during labour enters hospital in labour, she should be approached at the earliest opportunity to reaffirm her consent to participate in the study. This should be prior to the administration of any other drugs.

Such a scheme for obtaining consent to participation in a research project during labour will be acceptable to some (and hopefully, most) research ethics committees, but each individual committee will have its own view and researchers should seek local advice on this matter.

The imperative to publish results

If a study has been appropriately designed and conducted, there is likely to be an outcome worthy of publication. Whether publication is easy or only occurs after repeated submissions may be influenced by the results. If a study shows a clear difference between two drugs or treatment regimens, and the study was well designed and properly conducted, then the findings are more likely to be published. If, however, the findings suggest no difference between two drugs or treatments, publication, though just as important, may not be as easy. The overriding principle must be that if the study was conducted in a proper manner, the results should be made available to the medical world, even if the results are contrary to expectations and, hence, rather disappointing. It is shameful that, in the past, results have been withheld when they have not been supportive of the new drug or treatment.

The ethical imperative to publish is based in the conditions under which the patient consents to participate, namely, the general good of research per se. If a patient or volunteer is prepared to enter a study to further this good (and irrespective of the trial outcome or any personal benefits that they may have derived, it should be remembered that they have already taken the risks), there must be a duty to ensure that the information obtained is used and not kept secret.

It is unfortunate that many studies that are submitted for publication are rejected because of poor study design or poor conduct of the study. Whilst it is the researcher's responsibility to design a study that will ensure an unbiased assessment of the subject under investigation, there is also a responsibility on others, such as the LRECs/MRECs, to check study design prior to the research project starting. For the same reason that it unethical not to publish, it is un-ethical to undertake a research project that is so badly designed that it cannot produce any reliable results.

Journals have an important role to play in supporting ethical research practice by refusing to consider papers for publication unless the authors can guarantee appropriate and prospective ethical approval. All the main English-language anaesthetic journals state this in their 'Instructions to Authors', though sadly some investigators fail to meet this requirement. The editorial board of a journal may be faced with the unenviable task of rejecting a major research finding because the authors have failed in this most fundamental of requirements.

In defence of the researcher seeking publication, it can be very confusing because, even if ethics committee approval has been obtained, a particular jour-nal may have the opinion that the work does not reach the required ethical stan-dards – either as a consequence of the country of origin's interpretation of the ethical issues, or concerns over whether all information was provided to the research ethics committee when it considered the application. This may seem a somewhat 'high-handed' approach from any particular journal, but one has to remember that the editor of a scientific journal has a responsibility to ensure that any research material published has been conducted properly, both scientifically and ethically.

Case reports – research or observation?

The case report has been a major contributor to the development of modern anaesthetic practice, and it has often been the catalyst for an extensive research project. Most case reports fall into one of the following categories: an interesting syndrome posing particular anaesthetic challenges; a use of a drug for a different purpose than that for which it has a licence; or an unexpected incident and its management.

It might seem that these are perfectly simple observations of clinical practice and, therefore, of no research or ethical interest but, as in other areas of publica-tion, the ground is moving and case reports are now receiving much closer ethi-cal scrutiny. The class of case report giving the greatest ethical concern is the use of a drug outside its licensed indication, particularly when a licensed substance was available. An example might be the reported use of an opioid-like drug administered into the epidural space. Whilst there are no opioids licensed for epidural administration, extensive clinical experience with some (fentanyl, diamorphine) has conferred an element of safety and 'normal practice'. To use a hitherto unused alternative on a one-off basis may be interesting but it is certainly not ethical when a perfectly acceptable alternative was available.

Another ethical aspect of case reports pertains to the identity of the subject. In the recent past, there have been incidences where patients have been recognised (despite obscuring features in any photographs). This has led most anaesthetic journals to require consent from the patient (or assent from the family if obtaining consent is inappropriate or impossible) for the publication of, what is, their personal information.

Conclusion

It is now widely accepted that medical research must only be undertaken with full consideration of any ethical issues. Research ethics committees have a role in ensuring that research protocols are ethically acceptable. Clinicians should ensure that research is not conducted inadvertently in the form of audit or case reports. Medical journals are becoming ever more concerned over ethical issues surrounding submitted manuscripts. Meticulous attention to detail in dealing with ethical matters in clinical studies will not only ensure good quality research, but it will also ensure the continuing support and trust of the public, which is so necessary for the future of clinical research.

References

1. General Medical Council. Research: The roles and responsibilities of doctors. London: GMC, 2000
2. World Medical Association Declaration of Helsinki: Ethical principles for medical research involving human subjects. Adopted Helsinki, 1964; amended Edinburgh, 2000. Available at: www.wma.net
3. Wilson AJ, Diemunsch P, Lindeque BG, et al. Single-dose i.v. granisetron in the prevention of postoperative nausea and vomiting. Br J Anaesth 1996; 76: 515–18
4. Fujii Y, Tanaka H, Kawasaki T. Pre-operative oral granisetron for prevention of postoperative nausea and vomiting after breast surgery. Eur J Surg 2001; 167: 184–7
5. Anon. A Charter for Ethical Research in Maternity Care. Association for Improvements in the Maternity Services, The National Childbirth Trust and the Maternity Alliance, 1997 [http://ourworld.compserve.com/homepages/Bulletin-of-Medical-Ethics/charter.htm]

Recommended Reading

General Medical Council Research. The role and responsibilities of doctors. London: GMC, 2000
General Medical Council. Seeking patients' consent: the ethical considerations. London: GMC, 1999
Medical Research Council. Guidelines for Good Clinical Practice in Clinical Trials. London: MRC, 1998
Anon. Investigators. Anaesthesia and ethics [Editorial]. Anaesthesia 2000; 55: 521–2

Research Ethics 8

Richard Nicholson

Introduction – the development of protection for research subjects

Controls on the conduct of medical research, in order to protect its human subjects, have developed in a fairly consistent pattern. First, a medical researcher oversteps the limit of what is acceptable in his society, damages or kills the research subjects, and causes a scandal. Then the authorities respond to the ensuing public outcry by writing new laws and regulations. It is a pattern seen on several occasions and in different countries.

The first example was in Prussia at the turn of the nineteenth century. Professor Neisser, working in Breslau, thought he had developed a vaccine against syphilis, but instead gave the disease to a number of young women. He was taken to court and fined the equivalent of two-thirds of his annual salary, and early in 1900 the Prussian Minister for Religious, Educational and Medical Affairs issued a directive on the conduct of medical research[1]. It was quite simple, saying, in effect, that medical research interventions could only be carried out on people who had given their unambiguous consent, after being warned of any possible negative consequences. Such interventions were only to be carried out by the medical director of the hospital or clinic, or with his authorisation.

It is not clear that the directive had much effect in practice. By the late 1920s, another scandal was brewing in Berlin, where an active chemical industry developed several potentially therapeutic substances but tested them in ways that put patients at considerable risk. As a result, the German Minister of the Interior issued regulations in 1931 that contain most of the elements we would now expect to see in regulations to control medical research[2]. Within less than a decade, however, one saw how little effect such regulations may have when the prevailing social ethos does not support them. They remained in force until 1945, but in no way deterred the doctors who atrociously misused concentration camp prisoners in pseudo-scientific experiments, costing hundreds of lives without providing any reliable or useful new knowledge.

One response to the Nazi experiments was again to write new guidelines. In this case they were written in 1947 as part of the judgment of the military tribunal on over 20 of the doctors involved, and became known as the Nuremberg Code. Like its predecessors, the Code was largely ignored: British and American doctors thought that it only applied to 'nasty Nazis' and could not possibly apply to them. Yet Nazi experiments in mass sterilization of women by using X-rays were probably based on the work of a New York gynaecologist[3], and, in 1946, two British doctors researched German babies to death[4]. This caused so little concern that one of them was elected a Fellow of the Royal Society within two years.

The pattern has continued. Revelations in 1972 about the Tuskegee syphilis study, in which hundreds of poor black men in Alabama were denied effective treatment for syphilis for 40 years[5], led to the passing of the US National Research Act[6]. Unethical and dangerous studies on babies in Stoke-on-Trent in the early 1990s led to the development in the UK of both research governance and new governance arrangements for research ethics committees[7,8].

What is not clear is how effective laws and regulations are when they are not developed by researchers and, consequently, are unlikely to be 'owned' by them. Such doubts have not, however, deterred those who like to write guidelines whether or not there has been a recent scandal. The number of guidelines is growing exponentially, with more than 20 new guidelines, regulations or directives in the last decade that are relevant in the UK.

One area in which there is a surprising absence of guidelines is anaesthetic research: the only recent guidance is on the conduct of obstetric anaesthetic research[9]. The gap is surprising because anaesthetics and anaesthetists have contributed their quota of scandalous experiments, thereby helping the development of research ethics.

The very first public demonstration of anaesthesia led to a scandal. William Morton demonstrated 'Letheon' at the Massachusetts General Hospital in October 1846 and, at first, kept secret its active ingredient. It is not clear whether his motive was to perfect the technique before revealing that he was using diethyl ether, or to try to control the supply of ether. Despite the successful demonstrations, surgeons at the hospital declined to use Letheon until told what was in it, and some attacked him for his secrecy. He soon capitulated, having provided an early example of the need for openness, to colleagues as well as to research subjects, in medical research[10].

Setting up ethics review committees

Committees to provide prior review of proposed research studies began to be set up in an ad hoc fashion in the United States in the 1950s. At first, most of them were made up of physicians only, but a paper by Henry Beecher[11], professor of research in anaesthesia at Harvard, helped to initiate a rapid expansion of such committees in Europe as well as the US, and a broadening of their membership. In 1966, he published a study of examples of unethical research that had, nevertheless, been published in leading American medical journals. The 22 examples he published included an example of anaesthetic research, described thus:

> This study of cyclopropane anesthesia and cardiac arrhythmias consisted of 31 patients. The average duration of the study was three hours, ranging from two to four and a half hours. 'Minor surgical procedures' were carried

out in all but one subject. Moderate to deep anesthesia, with endotracheal intubation and controlled respiration, was used. Carbon dioxide was injected into the closed respiratory system until cardiac arrhythmias appeared. Toxic levels of carbon dioxide were achieved and maintained for considerable periods. During the cyclopropane anesthesia a variety of pathological cardiac arrhythmias occurred. When the carbon dioxide tension was elevated above normal, ventricular extrasystoles were more numerous than when the carbon dioxide tension was normal, ventricular arrhythmias being continuous on one subject for ninety minutes. (This can lead to fatal fibrillation.)

Beecher's paper caused considerable uproar, mirrored a year later in the UK by Maurice Pappworth's book *Human Guinea Pigs*[12]. The US Public Health Service decided the same year, 1966, to require all research that it funded to have prior review by an ethics committee[13]. As a result, the first research ethics committees were established in Europe, and they were soon followed by others to try to prevent the sorts of unethical research listed by Beecher and Pappworth. Whereas ethics review of all federally funded medical research in the US was mandated by the 1974 National Research Act, in the UK there has been official encouragement, but no supporting law or regulations. It was the Royal College of Physicians of London that took ethics review seriously and published increasingly detailed guidelines between 1967 and 1996 on how research ethics committees should operate[14].

Central to that advice has been the requirement that research on human subjects should conform to the World Medical Association's Declaration of Helsinki[15]. The World Medical Association (WMA) was set up in 1947 as one response to the Nazi doctors' atrocities: it was to provide mutual, and international, support to doctors to maintain the highest ethical standards in their work. It soon realised that guidance on the conduct of research was necessary, since the Nuremberg Code, with its stark opening statement – 'The voluntary consent of the human subject is absolutely essential' – was proving difficult for research physicians to accept. After 12 years in preparation, the WMA's statement was agreed upon at its annual meeting in Helsinki in 1964.

The Declaration, through various revisions, has continued to be centred on the principle that the interests of the individual subject always take precedence over the interests of science and society. The latest version, agreed unanimously by 44 national medical association members of the WMA in Edinburgh in 2000, has aroused considerable controversy. It maintains the centrality of that principle, but expands on what it means in practice for how researchers must behave towards research subjects. Following it, and in particular its limitations on the use of placebo-controlled studies of new drugs, makes some research of dubious merit more difficult to do, leading to loud objections from the pharmaceutical industry and drug licensing authorities. It is important to remember, however, that the Declaration provides guiding ethical principles, written by doctors as a standard to which physician researchers worldwide should aspire. Just like the work of ethics review committees, it is not there to make life easy for researchers.

The role and function of research ethics committees

Neither, on the other hand, are ethics review committees supposed to make life hard for researchers. Their main purpose is to ensure that all proposed research can be carried out ethically, and to reassure the public that that is the case. To do so, they must satisfy themselves on various points:

- that the research is well-designed, and is capable of answering the question posed
- that the researchers are competent
- that putative subjects will be adequately informed in order to give their voluntary, informed consent
- that the potential benefits of the research are proportionate to the risks
- that subjects of the research will be selected equitably
- that there are adequate arrangements in place to compensate any subjects who may be harmed by the research[16].

How well they succeed in fulfilling that purpose is moot. Few genuinely unethical research projects are approved on either side of the Atlantic but many projects could be done better, and sometimes committees fail to recognise this. The problem for UK research ethics committees (RECs) is that, although most have been set up within the National Health Service, the Department of Health has never specifically made funds available either for training REC members and administrators, or to provide administrative support. By the early 1980s, over 250 RECs were in existence, with a wide variety of methods of working and of standards of review[17].

As larger, multicentre, studies became more common from the late 1980s onwards, the discrepancies between RECs became more obvious. Organisers of multicentre studies complained that different committees came to widely varying conclusions, wanted different changes to protocols, and were sometimes ridiculously slow in giving their opinion. As a rough rule of thumb, if a researcher approached more than 30 RECs, it would take over a year to obtain responses from all of them. While such delays were generally inexcusable, the variety of conclusions and changes requested is more readily understood. Almost any application to an REC is likely to have at least six to eight points that raise ethical issues. Given the highly variable levels of REC training, some may only pick up on one or two points, some may pick up on a range or combinations of the points, and a few may pick them all up. So wide variation in the responses to researchers is inevitable. However, it is also true to say that a few committees have delighted in unnecessary nit-picking.

In the mid-1990s, the Department of Health responded to complaints about REC performance by setting up ten multicentre research ethics committees (MRECs). Any researcher wishing to carry out a study in more than five NHS districts could go to any MREC to obtain ethical approval. This still had to be ratified by the local research ethics committee (LREC) in each district where the study was to be run, but it was only to consider local issues, and could have a small sub-committee do so. The local issues were whether the researcher was suitable, whether the local facilities were adequate, and whether the local population of potential research subjects was an appropriate one. With MRECs working to a regular monthly timetable of meetings, and LRECs required to respond within 21 days, it was expected that obtaining approval for a study would become much easier.

Unfortunately it did not. It took the MRECs a couple of years to establish the uniformity of speed and approach expected from the start. Initially, some MREC decisions were taking 5–6 months, instead of the maximum of two months originally envisaged. Many LRECs objected to having a new system imposed and continued to undertake full reviews. While the situation has improved, it remains rare for LRECs to consider local issues within the 21 days envisaged, and delays of three months remain common[18].

This is perhaps unsurprising. While the MREC system was set up with adequate staffing, funding and training, at the time of writing there has still been no move from the Department of Health, or the Central Office for Research Ethics Committees (COREC), to improve support for LRECs. Instead there has been the introduction of new governance arrangements for RECs, which have increased LREC workloads[8].

The governance arrangements for RECs, known as GAFREC, came partly into force during 2002. They provide much more detailed rules on how RECs are to work than any previous Department of Health guidance. In some ways this was necessary to reduce the variation between committees, which was demonstrated again in a recent study of LREC annual reports[19]. Just among teaching hospitals in England, there was one LREC whose chairman approved more than half the submissions before the committee saw them; another allowed just two members to review each proposal and, if they were happy, it was not seen by the rest of the committee; at a third teaching hospital, proposals submitted by LREC members had a 92% chance of approval without any modification, while those of non-members had only a 33% chance. It may be that members knew better what the committee required, and that there was no bias, but an impression of bias was inevitable.

GAFREC makes clear to whom committees are accountable, what research they must review, how the committee is to be set up and how it operates. It lays duties on members to attend a minimum number of meetings and also to undertake regular training. Decisions on proposals have to be made at a full committee meeting, the quorum for which is now defined in terms of the number of expert and lay members who must be present. Proposals on which a committee member is named must be reviewed by a different committee. The timescales for review are defined, so as to be in accord with the requirements of the European Union Clinical Trials Directive[20], which has to come into force as part of British law by May 2004.

One part of GAFREC that will affect all researchers is the introduction of a common application form for all RECs. It is a development from that used by MRECs, which has proved very useful, not only in requiring applicants to give all the information an REC needs, but also in giving clues as to the applicant's attitude to the proposal. There is a question asking what ethical problems the

111

investigator foresees. If the answer is none, or something trite and superficial, the committee is likely to take a long, hard look at the proposal, since often major ethical issues have not been recognised by the investigator.

It remains to be seen what will be the effect of GAFREC. As parts of it have come into force with no additional local support, a handful of experienced REC administrators has already left for less-onerous work. As REC members become aware of the increased duty to attend meetings and training, some too may leave. Doing the work of an REC thoroughly generally requires the voluntary commitment of at least 150 hours per annum. A greater danger of over-regulation, however, has been seen in the United States. The federal regulations are so detailed as to how research is to be conducted, and how institutional review boards (IRBs) – the US equivalent of RECs – are to function, that IRB members sometimes complain that they have no time to consider the ethics of proposals. They just concentrate on whether the research, and their consideration of it, falls within the regulations.

Informing patients about research

One part of every application to an REC, not on the application form, is the patient information sheet (PIS). This contains the minimum information to be provided to potential research subjects before they are asked for their consent to enter a study. The sheets are uniformly poor. A recent study of those received by the London MREC showed that 95% had been returned to investigators to be rewritten[21].

The most common problem is that investigators do not take the PIS seriously. Most of those submitted are a first draft written no more than two days before submission to the REC. Many now follow the advice of the Patient Information Sheet Working Party[22], and set out the information in a question and answer format. But the language used remains too technical, and the words and sentences too long. One PIS submitted to the London MREC by an eminent professor had an opening sentence of 93 words. Opening sentences in tabloid newspapers – the readability level at which one should aim – rarely have more than 20 words. Tables and diagrams are remarkable by their absence. When research subjects have to make several trips to hospital, with different tests or investigations each time, this information is much clearer in a table. Some investigators have never heard that readability diminishes rapidly with more than 50 characters to a line. In order to try to save pages, they print the PIS in a tiny font, with up to 140 characters per line.

The one thing that investigators could do, which would be most likely to speed approval of their research proposals, would be to write the PIS at least two weeks in advance. They should then give it to children in the 11–14 age range to read, and listen carefully to the comments. If they write for a reading age of 12 years, then over three-quarters of their potential subjects should be able to understand the PIS. At present, on average, the patient information sheets are written so that less than one-third of the population could understand them[23]. If reasonably intelligent children of 11–14 years – the investigator's own children, perhaps – cannot understand the PIS, it needs to be rewritten. What is quite inexplicable is that the average PIS submitted with proposals sponsored by the pharmaceutical industry is just as unreadable as those from academic researchers. If each company employed a tabloid newspaper journalist to write information sheets, they might save millions of pounds, since delays to clinical trials are reputed to be so expensive.

Equally inexplicable is the reliance, by almost all investigators, on just the PIS and an oral explanation. There is little knowledge of the large body of empirical evidence relating to giving patients or research subjects information, and to seeking their consent[24]. Yet it is clear that, as in education generally, the more often that information is presented, and the greater the variety of ways in which it is presented, the more likely it is to be understood. Some studies have only accepted as subjects those who obtain a perfect, or near-perfect, score in a multiple-choice examination paper. In preparation, potential subjects received, *inter alia*, lectures, slide shows, and self-assessment tasks, and almost all then passed the entrance examination for the study. It would add little to the cost of multicentre studies to produce, with ethics committee advice, videos or interactive computer programmes to enhance subjects' understanding of the studies. Much simpler interventions are also effective: one study showed that just adding one phone call from a nurse significantly improved subjects' understanding of a trial[25].

The principle that consent is only of value if given voluntarily, and by someone who has been adequately informed about the proposed research, has been in existence for over a century. Not only did the 1900 Prussian regulations require informed consent but, in the same year, Walter Reed acknowledged the principle by obtaining written consent from the subjects of his yellow fever studies in Cuba[26]. Obtaining informed consent assists researchers to uphold the fundamental principle of respect for persons. The importance of this principle in medical research is succinctly expounded in the Belmont Report, published by a US national commission in 1979, and available in many collections of important documents in bioethics[27].

How much information potential research subjects should be given remains a matter of debate. In recent years, guidance has become more specific, as seen in the International Commission on Harmonisation Good Clinical Practice guidelines (ICHGCP)[28], or GAFREC. In addition to the guidance of the Patient Information Sheet Working Party, Consumers for Ethics in Research (CERES) has published advice[29]. However, no statute law defines what information must be given, and there is still only one relevant piece of case law. Interestingly, however, it concerns anaesthetic research.

Walter Halushka was a student at the University of Saskatchewan in Canada. Trying to earn money during his summer vacation in 1961, he was told he could earn C$50 by being a research subject at the University Hospital. So he went to the anaesthetic department, where Dr Wyant explained to him that a new drug would be tried out, but that it was a perfectly safe test, having been conducted many times before. He would have electrodes on his arms, legs and head, and a catheter in a vein in his left arm. He needed to fast beforehand, and the test would take about two hours. He was not given written information, but signed a consent form.

The next day the procedure began as described. Then, however, the investigator advanced the catheter tip into the heart without telling Halushka. It caused some discomfort, and the investigator administered the anaesthetic under trial, which he had never used before. After half an hour, the level of anaesthesia appeared light, so more drug was given. Ten minutes later, Halushka had a cardiac arrest, was resuscitated using open cardiac massage, and remained in coma for four days. Thereafter, he was unable to concentrate, gave up his university course, and even found work as an electrician difficult. He sued the anaesthetists and the university, and was awarded C\$22 500. The judgment in the failed appeal by the university included:

> . . . There can be no exception to the ordinary requirements of disclosure in the case of research as there may well be in ordinary medical practice . . . The example of risks being properly hidden from a patient when it is important that he should not worry can have no application in the field of research. The subject of medical experimentation is entitled to a full and frank disclosure of all the facts, probabilities and opinions which a reasonable man might be expected to consider before giving his consent . . .

Although the appellant, Wyant, informed the respondent that a 'new drug' was to be tried out, he did not inform him that the new drug was, in fact, an anaesthetic of which he had no previous knowledge, nor that there was risk involved with the use of an anaesthetic. Inasmuch as no test had been previously conducted using the anaesthetic agent 'Fluoromar' to the knowledge of the appellants, the statement made to the respondent that it was a safe test which had been conducted many times before, when considered in the light of the medical evidence describing the characteristics of anaesthetic agents generally, was incorrect and was in reality a non-disclosure.

The respondent was not informed that the catheter would be advanced to and through his heart but was admittedly given to understand that it would be merely inserted in the vein in his arm. While it may be correct to say that the advancement of the catheter to the heart was not in itself dangerous and did not cause or contribute to the cause of the cardiac arrest, it was a circumstance which, if known, might very well have prompted the respondent to withhold his consent. The undisclosed or misrepresented facts need not concern matters which directly cause the ultimate damage if they are of a nature which might influence the judgment upon which the consent is based.'[30]

Issues in anaesthetic research

Such criticism as there has been of the Halushka decision by legal commentators has all been to suggest that there should be even stricter requirements for disclosure to potential research subjects than the appellate judges suggested. While that might be possible in the sort of research carried out on Walter Halushka, it is clearly not possible for much of the research that anaesthetists carry out when running intensive care units. Few patients requiring intensive care are in a position to take in information about research, let alone comprehend it or give a valid consent to their participation. English law, at present, gives intensive care researchers little help, since no one else may give consent on behalf of an adult with either temporary or long-term incapacity. The idea prevalent in some medical quarters that a physician may give consent to research on an adult with incapacity has no basis in law.

It is not necessary to argue here for the advantages of doing good research in intensive care to help to improve outcomes: the problem is how to do it lawfully and ethically. When patients cannot consent to a doctor's proposed interventions, whether by implied or explicit consent, the doctor's duty remains to do what is in the best interests of the patient. In research trials it is, therefore, important that there be equipoise – in effect an equal weight of medical opinion that either arm of a comparative trial might turn out to be best for the subjects[31]. This principle is of great importance when subjects cannot themselves consent. It is doubtful that a placebo-controlled trial of a new drug in intensive care, when there is already known to be an effective treatment available for that particular problem, would be held to be lawful in the absence of consent.

The Scottish law is ahead of that in England and Wales, with the section on medical research of the *Adults with Incapacity (Scotland) Act 2000* now in force[32]. Research on such an adult can be performed, provided that:

- it cannot be carried out on adults who could consent
- the purpose of the research is to gain knowledge related to the adult's incapacity
- it is likely to produce real and direct benefit to the adult
- the adult has not indicated unwillingness to take part
- the research has ethics committee approval
- the research entails no more than minimal risk
- it imposes no more than minimal discomfort
- consent has been obtained from any guardian or attorney with power to give it, or from the adult's nearest relative.

Doctors undertaking intensive care research in England and Wales would be unlikely to get into serious trouble if they follow the Scottish requirements when undertaking research intended to benefit the patient. The position of research not intended to benefit the patient (non-therapeutic research) is more difficult. The Scottish law follows the recommendation of the English Law Commission some years ago that such research is permissible provided it is likely to contribute a significant improvement of the scientific understanding of the adult's condition[33]. That provision has, however, been dropped from proposals to legislate on the Law Commission's recommendations in England.

Thorough review by an REC is vital in intensive care research, both to protect research subjects and to reduce the likelihood of investigators being accused of impropriety. The whole medical research enterprise is based on trust: RECs have to trust investigators to carry out research as approved, and subjects have to trust investigators not only to do just that which has been agreed between them, but also to do it with the highest possible level of technical competence. Such trust is dependent on openness, which was often absent in the past. As intensive care units developed in the 1970s and 1980s, it was rare for patients or relatives to be made aware of how much research was going on. It was thought that that information would just be an added burden. The presumption must now be in the other direction: that there will be openness about the research activities of the unit, and that it will require exceptional circumstances for information to be withheld.

While physicians, surgeons, paediatricians and psychiatrists all have official guidance on the conduct of research, the only guidelines available to anaesthetists appear to be those of the Obstetric Anaesthetists' Association[9]. They promote general principles of ethical research, but also address issues that arise because most research in this field takes place during labour. Various paragraphs illustrate this:

... 1.3 The welfare of the mother and the baby should always take priority over research aims.

1.4 The psychosocial and physical vulnerability of mothers (and their supporters/partners) should always be considered.

1.5 Multidisciplinary cooperation is essential. Investigators should always be sensitive to the views of midwives, obstetricians, neonatologists, general practitioners and other healthcare workers, who should be informed of the proposed anaesthetic research if appropriate. Investigators should also consider involving user groups or offering them information ...

2.4 It is strongly suggested that the process of informed consent during labour be witnessed by a practitioner independent of the research, e.g. a midwife or an obstetrician. This witness must be satisfied that the woman and her supporter/partner understand the study and its implications, and the right to decline without compromising her care.

One aspect of ethics review that may cause problems in anaesthetic research is assessment of the risks and benefits. The triad of anaesthesia produces sedation, analgesia and muscle relaxation. When potential new anaesthetic agents are introduced, these effects need to be assessed separately. Sedation and analgesia are often assessed in trials unrelated to anaesthesia and there are established protocols for doing so. Muscle relaxation is more difficult. Trial of a new muscle relaxant, or of the muscle relaxant effect of a broader anaesthetic agent, may require it to be given, without sedative or analgesic, to the point where respiratory muscle paralysis ensues and artificial ventilation of the subject while conscious becomes essential. Assessment of those risks is likely to give any ethics committee a major headache. Some years ago, it is said anecdotally, an REC struggled long and hard with whether to permit such a study. The committee finally gave approval on condition that the local professor of anaesthetics was the first subject, followed by the lecturers and senior lecturers in his department. They were in fact confident enough of each other's abilities, and of the safety of the new drug, to go ahead with the trial on that basis.

Conclusion

This rather discursive chapter has tried to show that ethical problems have been present since the earliest days of medical research. Two of the responses to this problem have been RECs and ever more regulations. They are based on sound ethical principles: most importantly, the duty to respect other people. From that principle is derived the overriding importance of informed consent, with the consequent need for investigators to think much harder than most currently do about how to ensure that their research subjects are adequately informed about proposed research. The difficulties of conducting ethical research on adults who lack capacity to consent, and the basis of all ethical medical research in trust, suggest that anaesthetists, in particular, need to be well aware of the requirements of research ethics before they take part in any medical research.

References

1. Vollman J, Winau R. The Prussian regulation of 1900: Early ethical standards for human experimentation in Germany. IRB: Rev Human Subj Res 1996; 18(4): 9–11
2. Reichsgesundheitsblatt, 11 March 1931; 10: 174–175. [English translation in Intl Dig Health Legisl 1980; 31: 408–11]
3. Mayer MD, Harris W, Wimpfheimer S. Therapeutic abortion by means of xray. Am J Obstet Gynecol 1936; 32: 945–57
4. Dean RFA, McCance RA. The renal responses of infants and adults to the administration of hypertonic solutions of sodium chloride and urea. J Physiol 1949; 109: 81–97
5. Reverby SM ed. Tuskegee's truths: rethinking the Tuskegee syphilis study. Chapel Hill: University of North Carolina Press, 2000
6. National Research Act 1974 (US Public Law 93–348). Reprinted in: Maloney DM (ed.). Protection of human research subjects. New York: Plenum, 1984, 23–30
7. Department of Health. Research governance framework for health and social care. London: Dept of Health, 2001
8. Department of Health. Governance arrangements for NHS research ethics committees. 2001. Available at: *http://www.doh.gov.uk/research/documents/gafrec.doc*
9. Obstetric Anaesthetists' Association. Guidelines for obstetric anaesthetic research. Bull Med Ethics 2001; 170: 8–9
10. Beecher HK. Scarce resources and medical advancement. In: Freund PA, ed. Experimentation with human subjects. London: George Allen and Unwin, 1972
11. Beecher HK. Ethics and clinical research. N Engl J Med 1966; 274: 1354–60
12. Pappworth MA. Human guinea pigs. London: Routledge and Kegan Paul, 1967
13. Memorandum of Surgeon General W H Stewart to the heads of institutions conducting research with public health grants. Washington DC: Public Health Service, 1966. Reprinted in: Katz J. Experimentation with human beings. New York: Russell Sage Foundation, 1972: 855
14. Royal College of Physicians of London. Guidelines on the practice of ethics committees in medical research involving human subjects. London: RCP, 1996
15. World Medical Association. Declaration of Helsinki: Ethical principles for medical research involving human subjects. Adopted Helsinki, 1964; amended 1975, 1983, 1989, 1996, and Edinburgh, 2000. Available at *www.wma.net*
16. Levine RJ. The value and limitations of ethical review committees for clinical research. In: Bankowski Z, Bernardelli JC. Medical ethics and medical education. Geneva: CIOMS, 1981
17. Nicholson RH, ed. Medical research with children: Ethics, law and practice. Oxford: Oxford University Press, 1986
18. News. Bull Med Ethics 2002; 181 (in press)
19. Godfrey E, Wray E, Nicholson R. Another look at LREC annual reports. Bull Med Ethics 2001; 171: 13–21
20. Directive 2001/20/EC of the European Parliament and of the Council of 4 April 2001 on the approximation of the laws, regulations and administrative provisions of the Member States relating to the implementation of

good clinical practice in the conduct of clinical trials on medicinal products for human use. Brussels: European Commission, 2001

21. Boyce M. Personal communication, 2002
22. Guidelines for researchers: patient information sheet and consent form. Available at: *http://www.corec.org.uk/wordDocs/pis.doc*
23. Nicholson RH. Unpublished data
24. Empirical research on informed consent: an annotated bibliography. Hastings Center Report 1999; supplement: s2–s42
25. Aaronson NK, Visser-Pol E, Leenhouts GH, et al. Telephone-based nursing intervention improves the effectiveness of the informed consent process in cancer clinical trials. J Clin Oncol 1996; 14: 984–96
26. Reed W, Carroll J, Agramonte A. The etiology of yellow fever: an additional note. JAMA 1901; 93: 431–40
27. National Commission for the Protection of Human Subjects of Biomedical and Behavioral Research. The Belmont Report: Ethical principles and guidelines for the protection of human subjects of research. Washington DC: US Government Printing Office, 1979
28. ICH guideline E6: Good clinical practice – consolidated guideline. Geneva: International Federation of Pharmaceutical Manufacturers Associations, 1996
29. Spreading the word on research, or patient information: how can we get it better? London: Consumers for Ethics in Research, 1993
30. *Halushka* v. *University of Saskatchewan* [1965] 52WWR608
31. Freedman B. Equipoise and the ethics of clinical research. N Engl J Med 1987; 317: 141–5
32. *Adults with Incapacity (Scotland) Act 2000.* Edinburgh: The Stationery Office
33. The Law Commission. Mental Incapacity. London: HMSO, 1995

Evidence-based Medicine and Anaesthetics 9

Lucy Frith

Introduction

There have been relatively few critical evaluations of evidence-based medicine (EBM). This is partly because of the novelty of the enterprise: it is only since the early 1990s that the term has had general currency, although the closely related 'outcomes based research' has had a longer history in the United States. However, another reason for the lack of critical gaze is that EBM appears to rest on an innocuous truism, a point amusingly made by a modern Socrates questioning Enthusiasticus, a supporter of EBM. 'I thought that all doctors were trained in the scientific tradition, one tenet of which is to examine the evidence on which their practice is based. How then does this new evidence-based medicine differ from traditional medicine?' (p. 1126)[1]. Evidence-based medicine does not differ from traditional medicine because it insists that medical practice should be based on evidence, rather EBM takes a different definition of what is good medical evidence and what are appropriate mechanisms for finding and evaluating this evidence.

The aim of this chapter is not to criticise the central premise of EBM – that medical practice should be based on some form of evidence – nor to question the nature of the evidence or the mechanisms for finding it. The aim is, rather, to consider how this evidence is employed in practice: how it affects clinical decision making. I will first examine what proponents of EBM mean by a better, more objective clinical decision, and then I shall show how interpretation and evaluation of the data are essential for applying the data in practice. Finally, I will examine the use of EBM in practice with the advent of best evidence clinical guidelines.

What is evidence-based medicine?

Fundamentally, the aim of EBM is to ground medical practice on good evidence so that the treatments patients receive are both the most effective and the least harmful. For example, the inadequacy of pethidine as an analgesic in labour has been well documented, therefore, on the basis of this evidence patients should not be given this form of pain relief[2]. In this way, patients, so it is claimed, will get the 'best' medical treatment based on the current state of knowledge. There is an implicit strand running through the literature that by using such tools in medicine decisions will be made on a more objective basis. Book titles such as *The Scientific Basis of the Health Service* conjure up images of a value-free Utopia. It is easy to suppose that as the evidence of effectiveness is improving and medical science is progressing we are increasing our knowledge base and thus decreasing the need for values. Medicine, in both clinical practice and research, is concerned with establishing the facts of the matter and scientific method is often thought to be defined by impartiality and objectivity.

> It is the objective nature by which the EBM paradigm approaches the question of 'what are we doing' and 'how can we do better' that causes health care providers and funding agencies to increasingly adopt this paradigm as a primary principle (p. 778)[3].

Evidence-based medicine has gained popularity due to an improvement in the standard of medical evidence. It is this improvement in medical evidence that is a crucial factor in the claim that clinical decisions can be made more objectively. Davidoff argues that, 'what has changed in clinical medicine in recent decades is the very nature of clinical evidence itself.'[4] According to Davidoff, the quality of medical evidence is improving by becoming more objective and, therefore, more reliable. Davidoff highlights three changes in clinical evidence. First, the standards for gathering information have altered. 'Case reports have yielded to population-derived studies of which the randomised control trial is the prototype or "gold-standard" of therapeutic evidence.'[4] Second, the means for assessing and interpreting clinical evidence has been expanded to include sophisticated concepts and techniques of experimental trial design, decision analysis and clinical epidemiology. An important element in this assessment of information is the belief that, 'the concept that a single study, although it might provide the truth, is often not enough. The whole truth may require a synthesis of the evidence from all the best studies, optimally through the use of meta-analysis.'[4] Finally, in the past, expert opinion carried as much weight as clinical scientific record. Whereas now, 'Authoritarian medicine may thus be gradually yielding to authoritative medicine.'[4]

An important element in this improvement of medical evidence is the use of systematic reviews. The reviews are a formal process to eliminate what could be termed clinical judgement: to replace a subjective process with an objective one for appraising clinical evidence. This process begins by the doctor conducting a systematic review of the research evidence and then combining the results of the primary studies to produce what is termed a meta-analysis of the results.

> Meta-analysis is a quantitative approach for systematically combining the results of previous research in order to arrive at conclusions about the body of research. Studies of a topic are systematically identified. Criteria for including and excluding studies are defined, and data from eligible studies

are abstracted. Last, the data are combined statistically, yielding a quantitative estimate of the size of the effect of treatment and a test of homogeneity in the estimate of effect size (p. 5)[5].

Mulrow comments that, although sometimes arduous and time consuming, this methodology is usually quicker and less costly than embarking on a new study[6]. This methodology can also be supported by the argument that it is more ethical to gather information from studies already done than conduct new ones and subject further patients to the potential risks and harms of a randomised clinical trial (RCT).

The most important aspects of meta-analysis are the criteria that delineate an acceptable study for inclusion in the review. The main criterion for the inclusion of a study in a systematic review is that it is a randomised controlled study. Although meta-analyses admit the use of other types of studies, these are often only recommended if no suitable randomised studies have been conducted. Once the relevant studies have been found, they must be evaluated against a predetermined checklist to ensure two main aims. First, that the studies have produced a significant result. For example, what was the size of the treatment effect; how precise was the treatment effect; and do the conclusions flow from the evidence that is reviewed? Second, that the study was methodologically sound. For example, were the procedures of randomisation adequate; and were the researchers blinded to the treatment protocols? If there are defined criteria then this, 'explicitness about how decisions were made enables others to assess how well the process protected against errors' (p. 76)[7]. Sackett, for example, argues that the important aspect of EBM is to make explicit non-explicit clinical reasoning[8]. Hence, the focus of attention is on the methodology of the decision process, and there is a belief that once this process is followed a 'better' decision will be made.

These claims, that clinical decisions can be made more objectively by using EBM are based on two underlying assumptions. First, that there is rigorous evidence available on which to base treatment decisions. It is presupposed that this evidence is objective in the ontological sense, that is, it exists independently of any perceptions people may have of it and, hence, is a more accurate picture of reality. Second, that by a clearly defined scientific process that is non-subjective and not open to individual interpretation, such as systematic reviews, it is possible to gain access to this objective evidence and, hence, use this evidence to make an objective clinical decision.

This is perhaps the idealised view of what EBM can offer medical practice: a dream of a value-free Utopia. However, there are two reasons why EBM cannot deliver this dream. First, there is often simply not the evidence available to enable all treatment decisions to be based on evidence from an RCT, and some interventions have never been the subject of a clinical trial. For example, in critical care there are a large number of interventions for which there is little evidence on which to base assessments of their risks and benefits: different modes of ventilation, the optimum fluid balance status of a critically ill patient and the use of the pulmonary artery catheter[9]. David Naylor argues that EBM is limited by the existence of large areas of clinical practice in which evidence is either lacking or

In the belief that it is possible to locate one best treatment or a range of specific treatments, it has been suggested that clinical guidelines should be used that are formulated on the basis of the 'best' evidence. Clinical guidelines are an attempt to introduce evidence-based practice at an institutional level, to ensure that medical care is evidence-based and everyone receives the best treatment. The formulation of protocols and guidelines removes the need for individual doctors to have to process the information for themselves by conducting their own systematic review. The NHS Executive has stated, 'on the advice of the Clinical Outcomes Group, [they have] begun to commend a selected number of high quality guidelines.'[18] These guidelines are to be used to inform the clinical management of various groups of illness. Protocols will be formulated by national experts in the field, who will be up to date and informed about the most recent research data and will have conducted the relevant systematic reviews of the literature. These guidelines are an attempt to provide a consistent package of care throughout the NHS, rather than allowing treatments to vary depending on the area in which they are given. The rationale behind guidelines is an attempt to both increase the quality of care and reduce the inequalities in access to health care.

The main problem with instituting national guidelines on a particular treatment is that patients respond differently to treatments, and the effect can differ from person to person. Guidelines rely on patient homogeneity, that is, on patients being very similar. However, in anaesthetics and intensive care medicine patient heterogeneity is high[9,19], and it is difficult to write a precisely defined clinical guideline. Even patients with identical manifestations of a particular disease could give different weight to various outcomes, depending on personal taste, social and family situations, life priorities and so on. When used to promote greater quality of health care, guidelines can incorporate an assessment of quality that is held to be the same for all patients. This could come into conflict with an individual's conception of desirable benefit and their own personal quality assessment. As argued above, even using the process of EBM, the data still have to be interpreted and an evaluation of how applicable those data are to the individual patient still needs to take place. In contrast, clinical guidelines trade on the belief that it is possible to establish what are the best treatments across the board. The concern here is that clinical guidelines might preclude an assessment of the suitability of a treatment for a particular individual. In the foreword to the Royal College of Anaesthetist's *Guidelines for the Provision of Anaesthetic Services*, this problem is addressed. It states:

> This document should be considered as guidance only. It is not intended to replace the clinical judgment of the individual anaesthetist; the freedom to determine the treatment of individual patients should not be constrained by a rigid application of the guidance. (p. 5)[20]

There are, however, areas where guidelines are more applicable. For example, the general guidance that the Royal College of Anaesthetists provided on patient information before day surgery is very helpful and sets out broad recommendations as to what information patients should be given to ensure that they are adequately informed[21]. Guidelines should not, however, be extended to areas of health-care provision where guidelines may be inappropriate. Even when patients are suffering from the same condition, guidelines should not be applied without thinking carefully about how applicable they are to that individual patient. It could be argued that, due to the individual nature of many treatment decisions, it could be very difficult to produce guidelines that reflected each patient's treatment preferences.

Many authors have drawn attention to the importance of recognising that good outcomes must be seen as relative to the patient. Hopkins and Soloman illustrate this point with the example of the management of stroke patients[22]. They say that the course of the treatment and the outcomes of rehabilitation cannot be predetermined because each person's disability is unique. Hence, the therapist has to concentrate on the goals and needs of the particular patients. An editorial on critical care outcomes[23] demonstrates the complexity of formulating focused well-defined outcome measures in this area and the recognition that, for the patient, outcomes are related to their experience of the whole of the healthcare system, and critical care may only be a small part of this. This illustrates that effectiveness should be seen as a relative concept: relative to the individual who receives the treatment.

However, supporters of clinical guidelines might argue against this view of the treatment process. They might argue that there are enough similarities between patients suffering from the same condition to see them as being members of the same patient group (in statistical language, forming part of the same reference class of patient). Therefore, all that needs to be established is which group the patient belongs to, and then the appropriate clinical guideline can be followed. Patrick Suppes, for example, has argued that a decision regarding the individual patient can be extrapolated from other cases:

> Even though patients may vary in many respects (age, wealth, etc.), the direct medical consequences and the direct financial cost of a given method of treatment are the most important consequences, and these can be evaluated by summing across the patients and ignoring more individual features.[24]

Suppes is right in one respect. It may be possible to construct broad generalisations about patients' preferences for certain medical consequences. However, these would have to remain at a very broad level as many of the individual factors affecting these consequences are ignored. Although it might be possible to ascertain the types of consequence that are, on the whole, most important, it is impossible to predetermine their respective value objectively. For example, let us imagine a young orthodox Jewish girl in intensive care. After formal brain-stem testing, she is declared brain dead. However, according to Jewish law the child is still alive and her parents refuse to countenance withdrawal of care as they feel that this would be tantamount to murder[25]. This case illustrates that patients' values and priorities may vary widely depending on the individuals involved and their circumstances. In this case, it would not be ethically acceptable to impose the Royal College of Paediatrics and Child Health guidelines on withdrawal of care[26]. In the light of the parents' views, a different care plan was drawn up: one that permitted the limitation of care to allow asystole to occur as rapidly as possible, without hastening the cessation of the heartbeat.

125

In summary, clinical guidelines could restrict a patient's ability to receive the treatment that is most suitable for them. One possible way of protecting the welfare of the individual is to ensure that the patient always gives informed consent to any procedure. It is ethically desirable to get informed consent as a way of both respecting the autonomy and safeguarding the best interests of the individual. To allow patients to make their own decisions about their health care – to respect autonomy – is one of the fundamental ethical requirements of medical practice. Consent is also one of the best ways of ensuring that the medical care given is in the best interests of the patient, as it is thought that the individual concerned will be the best person to promote his or her own interests. There are two elements of consent that can be usefully distinguished here. First, the information given and the quality of the patient's understanding of the offered treatments; second, the range of options presented to the patient. I shall concentrate on the latter. With the implementation of guidelines, the patient is only offered a choice between a limited range of options and, consequently, the choice becomes one of taking the offered option or leaving it. If the treatment that would most benefit the individual is not offered then consent in this context becomes a negative action, in that the act of consent can only be to refuse an option that the patient thinks is inappropriate or that they do not want. It is not to positively choose an option that may be most beneficial to the patient. Such a refusal clearly does little to safeguard a patient's interests because it does not provide the desired treatment.

Regarding these points, it could be countered that patients inevitably face a restricted range of options in any large health-care system. Therefore, when deciding what treatment is appropriate, both patient and doctor are constrained by the available options. However, the worry with the introduction of guidelines is that the limited flexibility that currently exists may be reduced even further. This is because the rationale behind guidelines is to recommend the 'best' treatment and to apply it to every patient. I would argue that there is no such thing as one 'best' treatment, rather the notion of 'best' treatment should be seen as a relative concept: relative to the individual patient.

Conclusion

As long as the contribution EBM can make to clinical decision making is realistically considered, with an awareness of the uncertainty that pervades medical practice, EBM can be an invaluable tool for clinicians. As an editorial in the British Medical Journal noted:

> . . . the information that is drowning us is biased. Whatever technique we use to try and reach the answers from the information – no matter whether it is a systematic review or grabbing the closest paper in the library – we cannot avoid that bias.[27]

Evidence-based medicine simply provides the information that is brought to bear on the decision – it is not the decision itself. This should be born in mind, lest the evaluative elements of decision making are obscured.

References

1. Grahame-Smith D. Evidence-based medicine: Socratic dissent. Br Med J 1995; 310: 1126–7
2. Aly E, Shilling R. Are we willing to change? Anaesthesia 2000; 55: 419–20
3. Cooper AB, Doig GS, Sibbald WJ. Pulmonary artery catheters in the critically ill: An overview of using the methodology of EBM. Crit Care Clin 1996; 12: 777–94
4. Davidoff F, Case K, Fried P. Evidence-Based Medicine: Why all the fuss? Ann Int Med 1995; 122: 727
5. Petitti D. Meta-Analysis, Decision Analysis and Cost Effectiveness: Methods for quantitative synthesis in medicine. Oxford: Oxford University Press, 1994
6. Mulrow CD. Rational for systematic reviews. In: Systematic Reviews. Chalmers I, Altman D, eds. London: BMJ Publishing Group, 1995
7. Oxman AD. Checklist for review articles In: Systematic Reviews. Chalmers I, Altman D, eds. London: BMJ Publishing Group, 1995
8. Sackett D, Haynes B, Guyatt G, Tugwell P. Clinical Epidemiology: A basic science for clinical medicine. Little, Brown, 1991
9. Wijetunge A, Baldock G. Evidence-based intensive care medicine. Anaesthesia 1998; 53: 419–21
10. Naylor CD. Grey Zones of clinical practice: some limits to evidence-based medicine. Lancet 1995; 345: 840–2
11. Muir Gray, J. Evidence-based Health Care: how to make health policy and management decisions. Edinburgh: Churchill Livingstone, 1997
12. Greenhalgh T. Papers that summarise other papers (systematic reviews and meta-analyses). Br Med J 1997; 315: 672–5
13. Rosenberg W, Donald A. Evidence-based Medicine: an approach to clinical problem solving. Br Med J 1995; 310: 1122–6
14. Pronovost P, et al. 'Evidence-based medicine in anesthesiology' Anesthetics Analgesia 2001; 92: 787–94
15. The centre for evidence-based medicine, Oxford: http://cebm.jr2.ox.ac.uk (accessed 12th March 2002)
16. The Secretary of State for Health. The new NHS, modern, dependable. HMSO, 1997
17. McBrien M, Winder J, Smyth L. Anaesthesia for magnetic resonance imaging: a survey of current practice in the UK and Ireland. Anaesthesia 2000; 55: 737–43
18. NHS Executive. Promoting Clinical Effectiveness: A Framework for action in and through the NHS. Leeds: Department of Health, 1996
19. Goodman NW. Anaesthesia and evidence-based medicine. Anaesthesia 1998; 53: 353–68
20. Royal College of Anaesthetists. Guidelines for the provision of anaesthetic services. RCA, 1999
21. Royal College of Anaesthetists, 2000
22. Hopkins A, Solomon JK. Can Contacts drive clinical care? Br Med J 1996; 313: 477–8
23. Ridley S. Critical care outcomes. Anaesthesia 2001; 56: 1–3
24. Suppes P. 1979 151
25. Inwald D, Jakobovits I, Petros A. Brain stem death: managing care when accepted medical guidelines and religious beliefs are in conflict. Br Med 2000; 320: 1266–8
26. Royal College of Paediatrics and Child Health. Withholding or withdrawing life saving treatment in children – a framework for practice. RCPCH, 1997
27. Editor's Choice. Doctors' information: excessive, crummy, and bent. Br Med J 1997; 315 (13 September)

Further Reading

Greenberg HM. Three threats to the capacity for excellence in medicine. Annals NY Acad Sci 1994; 729: 8–18.
Kitchiner D, Bundred P. Integrated Care Pathways. Arch Dis Child 1996; 75: 166–8.

Maternal Foetal Conflicts and the Anaesthetist's Role 10

Wendy Scott

Introduction

Anaesthetists who work in obstetric units have a responsibility for maternal safety and comfort. This work is performed within an ethos that respects the autonomy of the patient and the choices she might exercise. The presence of the foetus influences how the anaesthetist conducts anaesthesia, but the anaesthetist's first duty of care is to the woman[1], and this duty should not be overridden by the duty of care to the foetus. This chapter will look at some of the issues and potential conflicts that arise for anaesthetists working in this area.

Participation in termination of pregnancy

Section 4 of the *Abortion Act (1967)* allows individuals to refuse to perform or to participate in terminations if they have a conscientious objection. When an anaesthetist is looking at a prospective consultant, associate specialist or staff grade job, it is sensible to know what that job entails. Under an agreement between the Department of Health and the medical profession, job descriptions should indicate this fact if the post includes a termination of pregnancy service. If termination is part of the job description then professional intentions regarding abortion can be legitimately discussed at the job interview (and the same applies in obstetrics) (p. 167–8)[2]. Candidates cannot reasonably expect to be offered the job if they say at interview that they are not prepared to perform terminations (obstetricians) or anaesthetise for them (anaesthetists). If there is no mention of termination services in the job description then candidates cannot be questioned about their attitudes to termination. There is also agreement that trainee posts should not include termination services as part of the job description because experience in participation with, or performance of, terminations is not considered necessary for basic training (pp. 167–8)[2].

It is, practically, much easier for the rota-maker if an anaesthetist maintains the same view whatever the indication may be for the termination of pregnancy.

The *Confidential Enquiries* most recent report also notes:

> Every medical practitioner administering any drug is responsible for ensuring that the drug, its dose and method or route of administration is correct and appropriate. A request from another practitioner does not absolve him or her from that responsibility.[9]

This statement reinforces the view that anaesthetists are not technicians, and they should not jeopardise their own careers by giving drugs in doses they personally judge to be unacceptable at the request, or insistence, of another clinician.

Nor can an anaesthetist be ordered by a midwife to 'do an epidural'. A request can be made through a midwife but, if the anaesthetist believes there is a contraindication, the anaesthetist can refuse.

Tensions between the woman and medical professional

Responsibility in the context of maternal health is something that needs stating clearly and unambiguously. Health professionals do have duties to the woman, but a competent woman also has to take responsibility for her own decisions about her pregnancy and delivery. The principle of respect for autonomy is based not only on the right to make one's own decisions but also on the responsibility that one has for the consequences of these decisions once made. If a woman elects to have a home confinement having been given accurate and unbiased information about the risks and benefits then, should there be a complication either to herself or to the baby (about which she was told), she ought not to expect to win any claim of negligence against the hospital or any individual if, as a direct consequence of her own decision, she experienced a problem, unless, of course, there was subsequent negligence by the hospital.

Respect for the autonomy of pregnant women is now supported in common law where the rights of competent women to give or to refuse consent, even in the extreme situation of refusing to undergo Caesarean section, were upheld[10]. The medical profession has no mandate to work outside the law.

But there are tensions that go beyond any differences of judgement between a woman and her clinician. Maternal morbidity and mortality have continued to decline[11] but, despite clinicians' best endeavours to protect the well-being of mother and foetus, it is not possible to achieve zero morbidity and zero mortality. Advances in maternity care over the past decades have, however, given rise to unrealistic expectations for the service. This, in turn, may be responsible for the unprecedented number of complaints and claims against obstetricians, midwives and, to a lesser extent, obstetric anaesthetists when the birth experience has been less than ideal. The prevalent view is that if something has gone wrong then there must be someone to blame, but this may, of course, not be true.

Fear of litigation inevitably leads to defensive medicine and, partly, accounts for the increase in the percentage of babies born by Caesarean section[12]. Certain women, however, would prefer to have a Caesarean section rather than a vaginal delivery. Some obstetricians agree to such a request more readily than others, taking the view that it is her choice whether to have a section, providing she makes this choice in full knowledge of all the side-effects and complications. An anaesthetist is usually presented with a list of the names of women scheduled for theatre and the indication for the surgery is not discussed with the anaesthetist. A trainee anaesthetist would probably not question the indication. Consultants are more likely to discuss the matter with the obstetrician and to reiterate to the woman the relative risks of vaginal delivery versus operative delivery. An anaesthetist is within his or her rights to refuse to provide an anaesthetic if, in his or her judgement, the risks in a particular case (for example, morbid obesity or an allergy to certain anaesthetics) are too high given that the procedure is an elective one. The woman, however, is entitled to a second opinion, and it is good practice to refer her directly to another competent anaesthetist.

Elective Caesarean sections are now mainly performed under regional anaesthesia. In most units, over 90% of women have either a spinal anaesthetic or a combined spinal epidural[13]. When an anaesthetist sees a woman who is scheduled to have an elective Caesarean section, the risks and benefits of both regional and general anaesthesia should be explained, one of which is that the block may prove to be inadequate. A graded series of measures can, however, be taken to help to alleviate any pain, for instance Entonox, then short-acting opiates and, as a last resort, a general anaesthetic can be offered. A woman's consent must be obtained for each of these staged increases in analgesia. It is up to the woman, and not the anaesthetists, to decide how much pain she is able to bear, or may be willing to bear in order, for instance, to actually experience the birth of her child. Likewise, given a favourable balance of risks and benefits, a woman may prefer to have the whole procedure under a general anaesthetic.

Regional anaesthesia has contributed to the reduction in maternal mortality[14], and it has become the accepted anaesthetic of choice for elective (and also many emergency) operative interventions. However, it has also given rise to a steady increase in the number of legal claims for compensation when women have felt pain during the procedure. The success of any claim for compensation may depend upon whether a woman was warned that the block might not be completely effective, as well as whether other measures were in place to relieve her pain.

Child patients

The increase in the teenage pregnancy rate means, amongst other things, that it is becoming increasing common to treat pregnant young women who are legally children as far as consent to medical treatment is concerned. The issues of gaining consent for children and from children, and dealing with a child's refusal of consent, are discussed in Chapter 6, and the general legal principles outlined there can be readily applied to obstetric anaesthetics.

Ethnic and cultural diversity

Most large obstetric units serve a diverse group of people, and cultural differences can give rise to different needs. Conflicts can arise when the anaesthetist's cultural views differ from those of the woman, and language difficulties can compound a situation.

People who do not speak English have the same entitlement to consent for themselves as those whose English is fluent, and it is good practice to provide an interpreter for anyone unable to communicate effectively in the same language as the practitioner. It is also good practice for the interpreter to be independent so that information to, and from, the patient is not filtered or distorted in the interests of any third party.

Cultural differences may arise. For instance, a husband may insist that pain relief for childbirth is contrary to the cultural tradition of his wife and refuse to allow her to be given an epidural, without giving her any chance to decide for herself whether she would like pain relief. It may be impossible for the anaesthetist to know whether this is a genuine cultural difference or the husband's own preference, but, either way, the woman cannot be treated if she dutifully obeys her husband and does not give consent.

An increasingly common problem for all clinicians is trying to accommodate patients, and their relatives, who insist that only women practitioners treat women patients. Out of respect for cultural difference, these wishes should be respected, but it is not always possible to provide both the right skill mix and the required gender simultaneously, so insisting on the required gender may put both the woman and the foetus at risk. The correct response to this situation is not always clear because, whilst it may be in the woman's immediate medical interests to be seen by a male doctor, the longer-term harm might be worse – for instance, rejection by, and divorce from, the husband and separation from her children.

A basic understanding of the main rights of passage rituals of religious groups fosters good relationships between anaesthetist and patient. For instance, when a woman is awake during a Caesarean section, it is common for the anaesthetist to talk to and reassure her. However, awkwardness might be generated instead if a Sikh woman is asked what name she has in mind for her baby. This is because names are chosen by randomly opening the holy book, the Guru Granth Sahih: the letter at the top left hand page will be the first letter of the baby's name. Other religions have their own ways and traditions of naming a baby and a woman might feel inhibited explaining such rituals at this critical time.

Conclusion

Obstetric anaesthetists have a duty of care to provide pregnant women with analgesia and anaesthesia that is safe and effective. Respect and understanding of women, their traditions and cultures helps the anaesthetist and other health professionals to give obstetric patients a fulfilling experience of childbirth, and one over which they feel that they (and perhaps their partners) have had some control. Women may feel cheated when their wishes and perceived needs have not been taken into account. The recognition of the right of a woman to make her own choices reflects the fact that the paternalism prevalent amongst obstetricians and anaesthetists in the past is no longer acceptable.

With these choices, however, come responsibilities. Autonomy has a price and that is the acceptance of complications that may arise as a result of exercising that autonomy.

Response to Scott

Heather Draper

Introduction

It is obvious from other chapters in this collection that anaesthetists, of necessity, have to be good team players. In an intensive care unit (ICU), in theatre, in accident and emergency (A & E), anaesthetists clearly share some of the burden of ultimate responsibility for a patient's best interests, without always being able to influence the decisions made by medical colleagues. As Scott shows, there is an additional difficulty facing obstetric anaesthetists: that of having not one but two patients, both of whom have (sometimes competing) interests that cannot always be kept separate or served simultaneously. Furthermore, anaesthetists have their own interests to protect.

The legal (and ethical) interests of the foetus*

There is no agreement about what the moral status of a foetus is. There is no time here to rehearse the various philosophical arguments on this subject, but views range from holding that the foetus has a status equal to (if not greater than) that of any other human being, to the view that the foetus has no interests and, therefore, no status that affords it any kind of right to life. In between are numerous positions, forming a complete spectrum between these opposite views. The legal position is no less complex, and, although people like to think of the law as more clear cut than the philosophy (but this probably amounts to little more than the fact that the law is written down and people have to obey it), it is not the case that the law adopts a philosophically coherent or consistent position about life before birth. For instance, it is true that the law does not offer us much in the

---

*For the purposes of this discussion, the term foetus is taken to mean the entity from implantation until birth, unless otherwise specified.

139

of that decision when things do not turn out as they had planned, despite being warned of the possibilities. Therefore, if a woman makes an advance directive (as opposed to a birth plan) she must accept that this is a serious and potentially legally binding agreement on both sides. Whilst I am wholly sympathetic to the view expressed by Scott that once in pain her decision might be a better informed one, I am also sympathetic to the anaesthetist who feels bound by the advance directive. This dilemma highlights another point raised by Scott in the context of relationships with obstetricians, namely that time spent preventing problems arising is time well spent.

As Scott has also argued, practitioners also have duties to themselves, one of which is a sense of personal responsibility for the consequences of their actions. As far as termination and infertility treatments are concerned, practitioners do have some legal entitlement to make a conscientious objection. This offers some legal clarity, but not necessarily ethical clarity. Whilst it is fair to say that the public would not want a medical profession who left their consciences at home, it is also fair to say that when a profession brings its conscience to work, this too can create ethical problems. For some practitioners, for instance, any kind of involvement in termination is unconscionable, including the referral of a woman to a practitioner who is willing to help. Practitioners for whom the balance between foetal life and professional obligations always tells in favour of foetal life may also feel unable to fulfil their legal obligation to offer assistance when the woman's health, or even life, is at grave risk. In this, and other contexts, it is difficult to argue that the practitioner's moral sensibilities should always be paramount.

As a partial and working solution to this problem, practitioners seem to draw a distinction between what they actively do and what they fail to do. This enables them to refuse to become actively involved in a termination, but, at the same time, not actively do anything to prevent one taking place. But even this thinking is ethically questionable for if abortion truly is murder then how can one, in good conscience, stand idly by whilst it takes place? The fact that many people who are opposed to abortion would also never actively prevent one occurring suggests that even those opposed to abortion are not certain of the extent to which their own views ought to define the actions of others. If so, then the law regarding abortion in the UK is a workable compromise that most of us can live with, despite its lacking ethical clarity.

Whilst consent is required before any intervention takes place, it is also the case that practitioners are not obliged to do something just because it is what the woman herself wants (see for instance here Scott's discussion of elective Caesarean section). Consent is a patient's protection against unwanted interference with bodily integrity (or, in legal terms, trespass against the person or battery). It protects the freedom from interference rather than providing an active right to something. Therefore, the fact that a person is willing to consent to something does not give them an entitlement to that thing. Entitlement is a complex concept and related (amongst other things) to justice. It is wrong to deny one woman access to a procedure that a similar woman in the same health system is given, resources permitting. This is because she is entitled to be treated equally, and not necessarily because either of them have an inherent right to the procedure (though in some circumstances they may have). For this reason, practitioners do have to defend a refusal to treat, but from a position of its being reasonable for them to exercise judgement in the first place: it is a proactive rather than reactive sort of defence. Likewise, the law is correct to put the burden of proof for conscientious objection squarely on the shoulders of the objector. He or she must prove that this objection exists and that they have not refused to participate on the basis of some whim or personal prejudice against the woman concerned.

Clearly, patients also have responsibilities[17], and these extend to not making unreasonable demands on practitioners. The difficulty, however, lies in determining what counts as unreasonable in a given context. Is it unreasonable for a woman to seek help from a professional dedicated to preserving life and health when the help she wants will endanger the life or health of another? But even this question begs that of whether the foetus is entitled to be considered as 'another', which takes this commentary around full circle.

One of the difficulties for all practitioners working with pregnant women is that this question has not yet been settled decisively. In practice, the value awarded to the foetus is relative to the person forming the judgement, principally the pregnant woman. The danger with the conscience clause, and the subsequent (and possibility artificial) polarising of views in the medical profession, is that issues about the status of the foetus may interfere with good relationships being formed with the pregnant woman that allow her to work through her own views of what is of most relative importance to her. Whilst it is wrong to coerce a woman into making a particular decision, it is perhaps also part of maternal responsibility – and professional responsibility – for a woman to be very sure about what she is doing, and this includes the consequences of her decisions. Helping her to arrive at a decision is also in her interests and, therefore, part of the professional's responsibility to her. My fear is that the division of the profession into those who do or do not value foetal life, or who are pro or anti a woman's right to choose, may lead to a curtailing of discussions that are actually necessary if a woman is to make the best decision she can, and truly consent to or refuse consent for what her clinicians recommend.

References

1. Knapp RM. Medicolegal Aspects of Obstetric Anaesthesia. In: Manual of Obstetric Anaesthesia, 2nd edn. GW Ostheimer, ed. Churhchill Livingstone, 1992
2. Lee RG, Morgan D. Human Fertilisation and Embryology: Regulating the Reproductive Revolution. Blackstone Press, 2001
3. Cheek TG, Gutsche BB. Analgesia for Labor. In: Practical Obstetric Anesthesia. DM Dewan, DD Hood, eds. WB Saunders, 1997
4. The Association of Anaesthetists of Great Britain and Ireland. The Obstetric Anaesthetists Association. Guidelines for Obstetric Anaesthetic Services. London: The Association of Anaesthetists of Great Britain and Ireland, 1998
5. *F v. W. Berkshire HA* [1989] 2 All EL 545
6. Scott W. Ethics in Obstetric Anaesthesia. [Editorial] Anaesthesia 1996; 51: 717–18
7. Brooks H, Sullivan WJ. The importance of patient autonomy at birth. Intl J Obstet Anaesth 2002; 11: 196–203
8. *Malette v. Shulman* [1990] 67 DLR (4th) 321
9. Royal College of Obstetricians and Gynaecologists. Why Mothers Die 1997–1999. The Confidential Enquiries into Maternal Deaths in the United Kingdom. London: RCOG Press, 2001
10. *MB, Re (Medical Treatment)* [1997] 2 FLR 426

11. Drife J. Reducing Risks in Obstetrics. In: Clinical Risk Management. C Vincent, ed. London: BMJ Press, 1995
12. Rao KB. Caesarean deliveries–changing trends. In: The Management of Labour. S Arulkumaran, SS Ratnan, KB Rao, eds. Orient Longman, 1997
13. May AE, Buggy D. Obstetric anaesthesia and analgesia. In: Textbook of Anaesthesia, 4th edn. AR Aitkenhead, DJ Rowbotham, G Smith, eds. Churchill Livingstone, 2001
14. Department of Health. Why Mothers Die: a report of the triennial Confidential Enquiries into maternal death 1994–1996. London: Department of Health on behalf of The Controller of her Majesty's Stationery Office, 1998
15. Seymour J. Childbirth and the Law. Oxford: Oxford University Press, 2000
16. Draper H. Women, forced caesareans and antenatal responsibilities. J Med Ethics 1996; 22: 327–33
17. Draper H, Sorell T. Patients' responsibilities in medical ethics. Bioethics 2002; 16: 335–52

Resource Allocation in Critical Care   11

Richard Wenstone

Introduction

Few clinicians who practice Intensive Care Medicine can fail to be aware of resource issues; allocation decisions are a day-to-day occurrence and usually well known to staff and patients throughout the hospital system. Concerns about health-care resources and their allocation are aired by the general public and debated in the media.

For clinicians, the term 'resources' has a broad interpretation that includes beds, staff (medical, nursing and professions allied to medicine), equipment and drugs. Any or all of these may be, or seem to be, in short supply at any given moment in time. Continuing advances in what is medically possible, the cost of these interventions and public expectations all conspire to produce the recognition that resources are limited. In addition, issues of resources and their allocation may act on two different levels: first, those clinicians with a managerial responsibility, such as an intensive care unit (ICU) clinical director, may have budgetary control and responsibility for prioritisation of expenditure as well as strategy, policy-making and implementation; second, there are the more directly patient-orientated issues, such as assessing appropriateness for admission (or discharge) and finding a bed, staff or equipment for a new admission.

All intensivists deal with resource allocation issues on a regular basis, and these issues are inseparable from their clinical management of critically ill patients. These common and recurring issues are explored below.

General budgetary issues

Clinicians with budgetary control will have to face the tasks of asking for greater resources from Trust managers, purchasers (Primary Care Trusts) or from their local critical care network. Assuming the budget will not meet the demand for care, and having been allocated a fixed budget, the difficult task of prioritisation begins. Adequate resources for opening a new ICU bed (for which approximately 50% of the costs will be recurrent nursing salaries) will only rarely be made available. More mundane tasks, therefore, become necessary, for example, deciding which new (or replacement) drugs or items of equipment should be purchased versus expansion in number of staff versus development of 'outreach' (see below). Deciding on the preferred course of action will typically be a joint decision amongst the ICU consultant (and nursing) body, but a particular Trust interest may significantly reduce any apparent freedom of choice that they might otherwise have. For example, a Trust's desire to increase its activity with respect to a particular surgical procedure or to establish itself as a regional centre may force an increase in ICU expenditure on specific equipment or drugs.

Naturally, the major proportion of any ICU's budget will already be accounted for in terms of fixed costs over which there is, in reality, no control. This can frustrate clinicians in their attempts to introduce innovative drugs and technologies. Indeed, one could label this whole process an example of health-care rationing and, of course, clinicians may well consider that this process has, for them, no real ethical issue attached. They may perceive resource allocation at this level to be divorced from their direct patient care and, therefore, someone else's responsibility. Clinicians may feel pressured into working with managers, and if they perceive any sense of conflict in this entire process it may well be with those whom they perceive as holding the purse-strings. Clinicians, divorced as they are on the whole from budget-*setting* processes (as opposed to budget-*holding*) may, rightly, perceive budgets as *imposed* rather than *agreed*. Any such perception is likely to be further exacerbated by the introduction of budgetary cuts dressed up as cost-improvement measures. Furthermore, the establishment or expansion of particular surgical activities, as noted above, may impact heavily on the demand for ICU resources. Such undertakings are frequently made without *prior* assessment of the demand and funding for ICU, thereby straining resources even further.

Undoubtedly, the allocation tasks most immediately felt by intensivists relate to their direct care of patients: the decision-making process around admission to the ICU, transfer to ICUs in other hospitals and discharge from ICU.

Admission policies

Clearly, it is neither possible nor desirable to admit every referred patient; for some, the prospects of survival would be vanishingly small. This, however, raises the question of how the likelihood of survival – and survival for how long – is assessed and if available space within the ICU should determine whether or not a patient is admitted.

The UK Government has shown interest in the process of admission to ICU for some time (perhaps fuelled, in part, by successive governments' perceived electoral vulnerability to media interest in lack of ICU resources). In 1996, the Department of Health (DOH) published *Guidelines on Admission to and Discharge from Intensive Care and High Dependency Units*[1] in an attempt to try to encourage clarity and the adoption of more reproducible standards. This was echoed four years later, in May 2000, when the DOH published *Comprehensive Critical Care. Review of Adult Critical Care Services*[2]. By implication, the Government's view was that intensivists were admitting inappropriately; specifically, that too many of the patients treated were not going to benefit from intensive care and so, by implication, would waste resources.

Having an admission policy is now both commonplace and sensible. It can help to produce some degree of consistency in decision making within a hospital, allow the process to be more widely discussed and endorsed in each hospital, avoid potential accusations of discrimination (against the elderly, for example) and reduce the likelihood of personal biases being over-influential. Despite this, the admission decision-making process is complex and responsive to a number of influences, some of which may be quite subtle; so whilst it is obvious that, as the Government document suggested[2], inappropriate admission is a waste of resources, it arguably oversimplifies a highly complex problem.

Scoring

Assessing the likelihood of any particular individual patient benefiting from intensive care is not an exact science. Numerous scoring systems exist in the field of intensive care medicine, but the majority of these were designed, and are used, to assess 'degree of illness' (e.g. APACHE, SAPS, MODS) or 'amount of resource used' (e.g. TISS-28) rather than to predict the likelihood of death. In addition, these systems usually require data collection *after admission*, not at the time of referral. In the case of APACHE II[3] – one of the better validated, more sensitive and more widely used scoring systems – a full 24 hours of admission is required before a valid assessment can be made. Furthermore, it is designed for use on a *cohort* of patients not on individuals. As with any such system, errors introduced by lead-time bias (i.e. influence on the scoring system of actions taken prior to scoring, such as resuscitation) diminish their value. Thus, scoring a patient to determine *suitability* for admission is not a realistic practical option for clinicians. (However, early warning scoring systems designed for picking up deterioration in ward patients and used to prompt referral to critical care outreach teams (see below) or ICU may offer some utility.)

If formal scoring, and an approach at evidence-based decision making, is not an option for admission policies then what other techniques do clinicians use to decide on admission?

Information

There are patients for whom an assessment can be made on the basis of published data. For example, a notoriously difficult group of patients to treat is those with haematological malignancies. Despite their often young age, some sub-groups of these patients are recognised to have 100% ICU mortality[4]. Experience, of course, is probably a major influence on clinician decision making and, where evidence is lacking, inevitably forms the core of the decision-making process. Evidence-based medicine may be perceived as having, at best, a minor role in a large proportion of ICU admission decisions.

Some decisions, however, one would expect – or at least like to believe – are made on the basis of published data *and* experience, for they are complementary not mutually exclusive. Perhaps the best example of this is the common problem of patients with end-stage chronic obstructive pulmonary disease (COPD). These form a patient group commonly referred to intensive care, who are recognised to have a predictably high in-hospital mortality and poor long-term prognosis[5]. Most intensivists are familiar with 'failure to wean' COPD patients, who finally succumb after a prolonged ICU stay.

On the other hand, *lack of information* at the time of referral in the case of, for example, the collapsed patient urgently referred from the accident and emergency department, may lead to a hasty admission and is, therefore, frequently a cause of what may be retrospectively labelled an 'inappropriate admission'. It is common when reviewing ICU admissions for audit purposes that some admissions are termed 'inappropriate'.

There are at least two types of admission to ICU that may turn out to be 'inappropriate'. The first is an emergency patient, where little clinical information is available on which to base a decision. If the critical illness usually responds to ICU treatment, and in the absence of any other contradictory information (such as an advanced directive refusing treatment), this patient may well be admitted. The second type of patient may be referred by an admitting consultant following deterioration on the ward. In this case, there is often more information available for the ICU clinician to make a decision. Whilst a ward patient may suddenly deteriorate, the ICU consultant and the ward consultant will often have the opportunity to discuss the case. At this point, it may be possible to decide whether the patient can realistically be expected to benefit from ICU treatment or not. If the patient is terminally ill, ICU treatment may be inappropriate even if it can offer good quality palliative care.

To date, there are no published data showing any effect of the increasing public awareness of advanced directives (living wills) on ICU admission. My own impression is that, although some patients will have expressed a verbal opinion to relatives (and, rarely, their general practitioner), their prior views are of more value *after* ICU admission rather than aiding the decision of whether or not to *admit* to ICU.

Likely benefit to the patient

At first sight, one might assume that patients who are too ill to benefit from intensive care (for whom admission could be considered medically futile) would automatically be excluded (a criterion that all admission policies would presumably advocate). There is no legal or ethical duty to undertake futile treatment (see Chapter 13). 'Benefit' is, however, an undefined and nebulous term. Intensivists generally use the term to mean 'can be expected to survive until discharge from ICU'; but patients, their relatives and indeed other clinicians often seem to have different interpretations. Long-term quality of life assessments in the critical care population are difficult to make and not supported by quality literature[6]. Referring clinicians will have their own expectations and experiences about their individual patients (and their patient population), and this may, therefore, be a source of potential conflict for intensivists. Requests to 'just take him/her to give him/her a chance and see how he/she does' over the first 24 or 48 hours, or whatever period fashion dictates, abound. Such requests, though, are generally not persuasive; the vast majority of patients admitted to ICU will improve or stabilise in the period immediately following admission, as might be expected once aggressive resuscitation commences.* However, *peer pressure* from one's hospital consultant colleagues will undoubtedly influence admission decisions, and such pressure may be especially keenly felt where iatrogenic events may have contributed to the patient's current condition.

There may also be pressure from a patient's family or friends to admit them 'to give them every chance'. Such opinions may be unrealistic (public comprehension of risk/benefit is limited, which is fortunate for the purveyors of national lotteries), but they are often intense, unrelenting and vociferous and undoubtedly influence clinical decision making. Of course, one could argue that a decision to admit a patient *solely* because of such pressure is treating the family rather than treating the patient (in my experience this is also true when decisions to withdraw therapy are delayed), but this may be a way of attempting to rationalise an action against one's better judgement.

It is not uncommon, however, for clinicians to admit patients whom they expect to die[7]. In some cases, clinicians may feel bound to admit patients whom they expect to derive zero benefit from admission if they perceive that there is no other suitable environment in which that patient can be accommodated. A common example would be a patient post-cardiac arrest in whom spontaneous ventilation could not be re-established. Whether one should admit such hopeless patients (as some undoubtedly will be, particularly if the patient's pre-arrest condition was poor, CPR was prolonged or the presenting rhythm was asystole or pulseless electrical activity) to ICU or allow them to die (i.e. stop manually ventilating) on the ward is often a difficult decision. It is, consequently, quite likely that some patients will be inappropriately admitted because there is nowhere else for them to go. Presumably, a dispassionate or actuarial view of this scenario would conclude that such behaviour was grossly wasteful of resources. However, clinicians and nurses who work in ICU often feel that they may be better placed than general wards to ensure a comfortable dying process. This highlights the dilemma between good management of resources and providing compassionate health care: compassion is frequently not cost-effective but it is undoubtedly in the patient's best interest.

Intensivists recognise that admission criteria are *not* consistently applied across all patient groups. For example, the patient with a disseminated malignancy who presents with respiratory failure secondary to pneumonia might not be admitted because they are not considered likely to benefit from intensive care. However, the same patient presenting with, instead, a perforated duodenal ulcer who then undergoes emergency surgery might well be admitted for ventilatory support.

---

*Analysis of my own intensive care unit's database suggest that only approximately 1% of patients die within a few hours of admission to ICU even though the ultimate ICU-mortality is closer to 30%.

That a clinician can quantify the patient's relative benefit (or lack of benefit) from ICU care in either scenario is doubtful. The most likely reason for admitting this patient with a surgical rather than medical referral would seem to be a practical issue of where to locate the patient. It also raises the issue about the appropriateness of treatment decisions made prior to ICU admission. Once a surgical route has been decided upon, post-operative ICU care is often necessary. The decision to admit to ICU is forced by the decision to operate and becomes outside the intensivist's control.

In addition, it is likely that a decision regarding whether or not to admit a patient may be influenced by available space within the ICU; the ICU may be full or it may have insufficient staff to accept another admission. Where clinicians feel that they can make a clear assessment of the appropriateness/inappropriateness of admission, this is unlikely to be a factor. Where, however, some doubt exists about patient suitability, it seems likely that that knowledge of the current bed status of the ICU may have an impact on decision-making.

The issue of obtaining a 'Do Not Attempt Resuscitation' (DNAR) order for a patient in ICU is common. It frequently becomes apparent that a patient's chances of survival have vanished and that further care would simply prolong the dying process. Such realisation normally provokes discussion of withdrawal of therapy (see Chapter 13) and, therefore, by necessity, a DNAR. However, DNAR may be discussed without a proposal (or agreement) to withdraw care.

The opposite issue to not admitting patients who are too sick to benefit is the admission of patients too *well* to benefit. Intensivists, when managing the typical 'closed' unit (one in which patients can be admitted only by agreement with the intensivists and not directly by referring clinician as is the case in 'open' ICU) recognise themselves as gatekeepers to scarce and expensive resources (ICU beds) and so will try to avoid admitting patients unnecessarily to an ICU bed if that patient's care can be adequately maintained elsewhere. The incentives to do so are great.

However, the ease and feasibility of avoiding admitting relatively well patients will depend on, amongst other things, the standard of ward care, the availability of high-dependency care, the likelihood of deterioration in the patient's condition and the ability to provide input into the patient's management (known as 'critical care outreach').

There is a common, but admittedly difficult to substantiate, view that the general level of nurse staffing and care provided on wards has deteriorated in recent history. Certainly, observations (such as monitoring respiratory rate), procedures (such as central venous pressure monitoring) and the management of certain diseases (such as diabetic ketoacidosis), which were once common on many general wards, have become increasingly difficult or absent in that environment. This frequently increases the pressure to admit patients to ICU who might well have been manageable on a ward, thereby, in time, exacerbating the problem of limited ward experience to cope with sick patients. This is frequently a potential source of conflict between ICU staff and ward staff.

At the same time as there has been an increasing demand for intensive care, there seems to have been a fall in provision of intermediate care on wards producing an increasing polarisation of levels of care between wards and ICUs.

One of the relatively recent innovations aimed at addressing this issue has been the provision of critical care outreach teams (CCOTs) as suggested by the DOH in 2001[2]. The primary role of these teams is to reduce ICU admissions. By supporting ward or high-dependency unit (HDU) staff in the management of sicker patients, it is hoped that these patients will avoid an ICU admission (and hence approximately £1000 [€1600] per patient per day). In the case of HDUs, the CCOT can also assist in the introduction of techniques of care or monitoring (e.g. non-invasive continuous positive airway pressure, non-invasive ventilation, arterial lines) that might otherwise not be possible outside the ICU. Coupled with the introduction (to wards and HDU areas) of one of the many types of early warning scores, it is expected that at-risk patients will be referred to the CCOT, or an ICU opinion sought, sooner and managed in a more timely manner to avoid an ICU admission. (CCOTs may also have a role in identifying those patients for whom a DNAR order should be discussed or who would benefit from input from a palliative care team.)

However, many clinicians working in intensive care are suspicious that funding for CCOTs (staff and equipment) will divert resources away from other areas such as ICU or HDU. Indeed, if CCOTs are to make an impact, they will be needed more than just during normal working hours and, consequently, staffing costs may become substantial because outreach is generally staffed by the most senior (and, therefore, the most costly) ICU nurses. There is also the added concern that ward staff may find themselves under even greater pressure to accept patients than they were before, on the promise of support from CCOT.

Admitting the patient

Once the decision to admit a patient has been made, the issue becomes one of whether or not a bed is actually available. Even 'bed availability' has an imprecise definition; frequently the limiting factor is the availability of nursing staff, not the actual bed. Traditionally ICU care in the UK has provided 1:1 nursing care. Although this is certainly not the norm in other developed countries and has been challenged here, it has been seen as a significant barrier to overcome. Some flexibility has always existed in those units that admit ICU and HDU patients (the latter traditionally having a 1:2 nurse:patient ratio) but many units admitting (or perceiving themselves as admitting) only ICU patients have persisted with 1:1 ratios even when particular patients do not require it. Attempts to quantify this have included scoring systems based on nurse interventions such as TISS-28[8], or more recent attempts at dependency scoring. The DoH has attempted to define patients according to the level of care that they require irrespective of their geographical location within the hospital[2].

Flexibility with respect to nurse:patient ratios is undoubtedly seen as a better way to manage resources, but it can easily become a source of conflict between nursing and medical staff. (Clear guidelines and objective assessments of patients' needs in *advance* of a crisis should enable this process to work more smoothly.) Proposals to manage the nursing resource more effectively by calling in staff when needed are arguably less workable propositions, unless they rely on agency staff. However, reliance on agency staff has a significant, and difficult to control, impact on ICU budgets. The experience, training and availability of agency staff vary so greatly that specialist ICU agencies have emerged to meet the need in both the NHS and the private sector. Even with this provision, ICUs may be unable to find the most appropriate staff for any particular shift at short notice. The use of agency nurses, although initially attractive, may lead to difficulties for those managing budgets and problems for those managing the deployment of staff.

Despite opportunities for flexibility, there are frequent occasions in which the only solution appears to involve transferring a patient to a distant hospital or the early discharge of another patient from the ICU (see below).

Use of resources once admitted

As clinicians have become more involved in financial issues there is, without doubt, an increasing awareness of the cost of therapies, whether it be the relative price of equipment or of drugs. This awareness has grown despite the claim of some clinicians – admittedly heard with less and less frequency – that such matters are irrelevant or not a clinical problem. Nevertheless, it is doubtful that any clinician would knowingly, *all other things being equal*, use a more expensive therapy in preference to a cheaper one. The problem arises where the more expensive one has *some* advantages over (or fewer disadvantages than) its cheaper rival – for example, the various analgesic and sedative agents available for use in intensive care. Clinicians may attempt to tackle this problem by adopting guidelines or policies regarding the use of the more expensive choice in an attempt to contain costs without agreeing – or being seen to agree – to suboptimal therapy. This strategy does have some logic behind it, and it has been shown to be of benefit in reducing costs in, for example, the adoption of antibiotic policies[9].

Having said that, there is probably very little, if any, attempt at resource limitation for purely budgetary reasons in relation to individual patients once admitted to a critical care area. Decisions to limit, withhold or withdraw treatment or instigate a DNAR order have already been discussed; however, these strategies, common as they are in intensive care practice should be (and are, in my experience) purely *clinical* decisions not *economic* ones. It is of interest that this view is not always held by the general public. Patients' relatives, for instance, sometimes express the opinion that they understood that decisions to withdraw treatment are made with financial considerations in mind. Interestingly, such views are almost always expressed *positively*, i.e. that doctors *ought* to include this factor!

Transfer

The decisions of whether to transfer – and whom to transfer – are difficult tasks regularly troubling intensivists. These decisions are necessary when the ICU is full; either because there are no bed spaces left or the remaining bed spaces are unstaffed. A policy of last-in-first-out (i.e. transfer the newly referred and accepted patient) seems logical at first sight. The 'last in' patient is often not actually 'in' the ICU, but is usually being cared for by ICU staff in the area of the hospital where they developed the need for ICU: the ward, theatre recovery or Accident and Emergency. However, this presupposes that the newest referral will not only be *fit* for transfer but that they are also the most *appropriate* for transfer. For example, clinicians will be unwilling to transfer a patient who is under the care of a specialist service not readily available in nearby hospitals (such as transplant surgery) to another hospital without that expertise. In addition to variations in availability of support services in other hospitals, not all ICUs can provide the same facilities (for example, renal replacement therapy or intra-cranial pressure monitoring), which the referring intensivists may feel is a necessary precondition before agreeing to transfer their patient.

So, should the patient, presumably already in the ICU, who is the most fit for transfer be selected instead? Such patients are often very recent admissions (e.g. following elective surgery or drug overdose) or long-stay patients (e.g. being slowly weaned from mechanical ventilation following an infective exacerbation of COPD). In both cases, clinicians – and nursing staff – may feel ill at ease with the idea of transferring these patients to make room for a new admission because they have a duty of care to their existing patients. Such stark realities may put pressure on ICU nursing staff to open another bed (assuming the last physical bed space was not already occupied) or put similar pressure on nursing (and medical) staff elsewhere in the hospital to accommodate the patient (e.g. the Operating Department Recovery Ward) even though such accommodation may be, strictly speaking, inappropriate.

Additional factors that influence the decision-making process may include issues such as attitude and mobility of relatives (a trip by ambulance to a nearby hospital may take 30 minutes but the same journey made by a non-car owning relative may require three buses and 90 minutes); sheer distance involved (not all hospitals have other ICUs within a reasonable distance); whether or not the patient has already been transferred (prior to their current admission); and even time of day (there is often a greater reluctance to transfer patients out-of-hours). Some receiving units may prefer a particular category of patient – for example, one who is expected to recover quickly, such as a patient requiring ventilation following a drug overdose. On the other hand, some ICUs may feel that *all* hospitals should be able to accommodate their own patients temporarily without transfer. Somewhere in the middle of all of this is the clinician's knowledge that rarely, if ever, is an individual patient best served by being moved anywhere; but what is in the patient's best interests, to undergo a long transfer to a proper ICU or be held, hopefully temporarily, in a sub-optimal environment? This balance between beneficence (trying to benefit the patient) and non-malfeasance (avoiding harming the patient) is a difficult one for all clinicians. If resources were unlimited, the issue would merely be one of appropriateness of admission, but where all admissions are appropriate with insufficient resources, clinicians need to have clear policies that can help them make consistent decisions.

In addition, the process of transferring a patient ties up at least two members of staff for at least double the time of the actual transfer. Although there is some interest in *dedicated* transfer teams[10], these are still not the norm. Depletion of hospital staff may, conceivably, place patients in the transferring unit at additional risk. The health and safety implications of the physical risk to staff involved in the unfamiliar environment of a transfer should also not be dismissed lightly.

Such a wide collection of factors inevitably leads to differences of opinion between different ICUs and, indeed, even within ICUs. Some ICUs may go to great lengths to avoid transfers, whilst others may choose more frequently to do so. These decisions may be further influenced by how important local clinicians see the need to keep down the number of transfers or, perhaps to allow them to rise (to support, perhaps, demands for more resources).

Political or financial pressures may also tempt local mangers (and politicians) to try to influence a particular hospital's strategy: on the one hand, transfers inevitably bring the risk of 'bad press' but, on the other hand, full recovery wards and ICUs run the risk of causing the cancellation of elective surgery.

Discharging patients

Given the issues involved in the transfer of patients, it is not surprising that clinicians will try to avoid transfers if space can be created within the ICU by discharging a patient. What this may frequently lead to is pressure to discharge a patient early – i.e. before one would, ideally, have wished to discharge them. This might be simply a question of time of day; there is a reluctance to discharge patients out-of-hours because, apart from the disruption to other patients (on the ICU and the receiving ward) that this causes, such discharges are associated with increased mortality[11] and risk of readmission to ICU. Clinicians will also be aware that evidence suggests that delaying discharge for 48 hours can significantly reduce mortality[12]. Alternatively, and more worryingly, there may be a genuine doubt about the receiving ward's ability (even if it is an HDU) or suitability to care for that patient at that time. Again, this leads to pressure on the nursing staff of those wards perhaps allayed, to some extent, by the promise of support from the CCOT (see above – though this may not actually be available out of hours).

Conclusion

Clinicians often face difficult decisions on how to distribute the scarce resource of ICU. They are under increasing pressure to make the best use of the resources they do have, and are censured for inappropriate admission. The fault, however, does not always lie with the ICU consultant, but rather it is a symptom of providing costly care for patients who receive little benefit in a health-care environment that is becoming increasingly cost conscious. There is a need for robust debate that engages health-care providers, purchasers and users, where policies can be made in line with available resources, and requests for increases to resources can be thoroughly analysed. The difficult decisions faced by many clinicians are often made in the middle of a busy shift and, frequently, in the middle of the night. Decisions made during these times and under these conditions are likely to be inconsistent and sometimes appear capricious. There is a need for decisions to be shared by all those responsible for providing and using ICU to ensure that both staff and patients benefit from appropriate use of ICU resources.

Response to Wenstone

June Jones

The provision of intensive care is very expensive. The Audit Commission Report on Intensive Care found that it costs six times more to care for a patient in an intensive care unit (ICU) than on a ward (p. 18)[13]. It is, therefore, not surprising that the Audit Commission recommended to the Government that cost savings should be made where possible. This responsibility is often devolved to those intensivists who take on the additional role of managing ICU budgets. This role brings with it an explicit requirement to make decisions concerning resource allocation, but this is an implicit requirement for all health-care professionals. When ICU staff are faced with resource allocation decisions, it is often in difficult or acute situations. Their task would be made easier if more consideration were given to how these allocation decisions should be made *prior* to an acute event happening. Some of the ethical considerations would revolve around identifying who ICUs should benefit and in what way, and how any risks or harms can be balanced against these possible benefits.

If a consultant is required to prioritise treatment between two or more patients, he or she will have many issues to consider, including:

- who will most benefit from the treatment
- what types of benefits are likely
- how long these benefits are likely to take
- the extent to which, when two or more patients need a single resource, any of them will be harmed by not receiving the treatment
- the extent to which, when two or more patients need a single resource, any of them could receive the treatment elsewhere.

The answers to these questions revolve around where the particular doctor places the balance between benefits and harms. There are specific ethical frameworks, most often used by health economists, that provide a calculus for making such decisions[14]. Clinicians, however, are likely to adopt a simpler consequentialist approach to balancing the benefits and harms. This approach, however, requires a decision to be made based on future outcomes, and predicting the future requires an element of guesswork. Given that failure to admit on to an ICU can result in a patient's death, admissions decisions made by intensivists are considerably more serious than they may be in other specialties. Indeed, the death of a patient may appear to be inevitable when, for instance, the ICU is full or under-staffed. At these difficult times there are a number ways in which decision making can be made easier by discussion between ICU managers and colleagues prior to crisis points being reached.

Access to treatment

When resources are scarce, those responsible for allocating them need to identify how these resources are most effectively used, a component of which will be deciding which patients should get access to them. Admission criteria are now perceived as a necessary tool for avoiding what has been termed 'inappropriate' admissions (and it should not be forgotten that 'inappropriate' applies equally well to those cases where ICU is *more* than is necessary as it does to ICU given in cases where there is little hope of benefit), but as Wenstone pointed out, admission criteria cannot always be consistently applied. Moreover, the existence of admission criteria implies that some patients should not be admitted to ICU because (a) they will not benefit or (b) their expected benefit is at too great a cost, either to themselves or the service as a whole. Health-care providers have often shied away from implementing admission guidelines because the consequences (death) are so serious if there is an error of judgement. It is impossible to completely eradicate error and, as Wenstone points out, admission may actually be necessary for an accurate assessment to be made. Where there is no immediate and local pressure on resources – for instance, where a bed is available – it is, therefore, understandable that staff may consider that it is safer (ethically, legally and medically) to admit the patient and treat them despite the doubtful benefit. This raises two questions:

- If treatment may be of limited benefit, should all patients be given a chance to benefit, no matter how small this benefit is?
- Should a patient who is unlikely to benefit from treatment be refused admission to ICU, even when there are empty beds?

The answer to the first question requires a balance between consistency and practicality. Because it is difficult to predict with absolute certainty how much benefit a patient will receive from admission, it is also difficult to assess the precise cost of any given admission, and it is, accordingly, difficult to make a true cost/benefit calculation. In terms of what is legally defensible, *where* the line (between 'sufficient' and 'insufficient' benefit to justify intervention) is drawn appears to be a secondary consideration. It is important that clinicians can show that they have drawn a defensible line within professional standards as per *Bolam*[15] and

Bolitho[16] where the primary preoccupation seems to be one of reasonableness, as judged through consistency rather than fairness in an absolute sense. Moreover, the process of judicial review is not only concerned with having guidelines and sticking to them, but also making similar exceptions to the general rule in similar cases. Given the fear that contemporary clinicians have of litigation, admission policies are more likely to be successful in practice if they are constructed in such a way that they provide the consistency that is required to defend decisions, if challenged, and the flexibility to identify and admit a deserving patient who would usually be refused, thus permitting a degree of room for clinical discretion. Whatever admissions policies are implemented, it is inevitable that admission in some instances will be deemed inappropriate because the likely risks and harms for the patient outweigh the likely benefits considerably. But, as Wenstone suggests, this leaves intensivists with two ethical problems: first, that admission policies are aimed at types of patients rather than individual patients and, second, intensivists have competing obligations to service the interests of individual patients on the one hand and to serve the needs of a patient population on the other. These two problems are brought into sharp focus when a unit only has one remaining bed. Is it right to give the last bed to a patient who is unlikely to benefit from treatment, especially when it is also likely that this bed will be needed, in the near future, by a different patient, possibly one whose potential to benefit is greater?

One way of addressing this problem is to consider whether it would be acceptable to give a bed to such a patient irrespective of the number of beds available, which leads to our second question of whether a patient who is unlikely to benefit from treatment should be refused admission to ICU, even when there are empty beds? (an increasingly unusual situation, because high bed occupancy has become the norm). Once it has been decided that potential for benefit is a necessary admission criteria, and, having decided the degree of predicted benefit that is required to justify the potential costs, for consistency's sake the availability of beds should not influence admission decisions. This means that a patient whose condition meets the criteria for admission, however marginally, should be admitted even if this uses the last bed, and a patient who fails to meet the criteria should not be admitted even if there are many available beds. The implied principle being consistently applied here relates not to the availability of particular beds on a particular occasion but to the just provision of intensive care in the round, namely that resources are utilised ethically only when they are used effectively because to use them ineffectively is to waste them. 'Waste' in this sense, does not refer to any value that the patient (or his/her family) might place on the resource, rather it refers to lost opportunity to gain the maximum benefit from the resource. Thus, whilst from the patient's point of view being given the opportunity of life, however small this is, is not a waste, when viewed in the round giving resources to such a patient is actually a lost (or 'wasted') opportunity to achieve greater good somewhere else. Irrespective of availability on a given day, ICU beds per se *are* a scarce resource.

Wenstone mentions that dying patients are sometimes the subject of inappropriate admission, his specific example is patients who are terminally ill. An ICU may be the only available environment for a patient to die with dignity when they have become biologically dependent on medical technology. If a compassionate view is taken, an ICU may be the best environment for this patient and their family for many reasons, but applying the principle that resources should be used where they give most benefit suggests that admission would be wasteful, particularly where benefit is associated with recovery. But this does not mean that terminally ill and dying patients gain no benefit from an ICU, rather they benefit in ways that could be achieved at less cost elsewhere. All dying patients need an environment in which to die properly – without pain, suffering or loss of dignity. Money may, however, be more effectively spent resourcing palliative care for patients highly dependent on technology rather than admitting such patients to an ICU. Unfortunately, such care is often either unavailable or thin on the ground. This raises two questions that there is no time to answer here. The first is how intensivists balance the competing obligations of compassion towards dying patients and just allocation of resources, given that the provision for palliative care is often inadequate. The second is whether intensivists should take a more active role in pushing for more extensive provision of palliative care as part of their role as gatekeepers to ICU resources.

Wenstone refers to two types of admission to ICU that may turn out to be 'inappropriate'. The first is an emergency patient, where little clinical information is available on which to base a decision. If the critical illness normally responds to ICU treatment and, in the absence of any other contradictory information (such as an advanced directive refusing treatment), this patient may well be admitted. The second type of patient may be referred by an admitting consultant following deterioration on the ward. In this case, there is often more information (and the possibility of discussing the patient with his or her ward consultant) available for the ICU clinician to make a decision.

It seems reasonable to differentiate between responsibility for accepting an emergency patient who later turns out to have been an inappropriate admission and a patient for whom the likelihood of successful ICU treatment was already extremely doubtful and known to the doctors involved. This distinction turns precisely on our having a greater responsibility for harms knowingly inflicted and harms unwittingly inflicted at times of crisis when quick decisions have to be made before all the facts are available. A similar kind of distinction is made when applying the legal concepts of necessity and duty of care. There is a standard duty of care owed to all patients, but, in an emergency situation, the doctrine of necessity permits clinicians to perform treatment for which they have no consent. Here, the law and common sense coincide, for, in most cases, it is clearly better for the patient to be treated without consent than to be left untreated and die because they were unable to consent. The law is unwilling to penalise a doctor for not having gained consent in these circumstances, providing there is no known objection to emergency treatment made by the patient whilst competent. The distinction between the planned or known and emergency seems to be a useful one to protect doctors from being held accountable for inappropriate admission in the case of emergency. If doctors knowingly admit a patient for whom an ICU is very unlikely to be beneficial and will merely prolong the dying process, then auditors will have some justification for claiming that resources are being used inappropriately.

Limiting treatment

Once a patient has been admitted and has received ICU treatment, a decision about whether treatment options should be limited may be required, and central to this decision may be the notion of futility. Continuing with an intervention that has ceased to have any therapeutic benefit cannot be justified when applying the principle that resources must be used effectively, and so such intervention must be withdrawn. (Arguably, such interventions cannot be justified for other reasons, discussed in Chapter 13.) Occasionally, treatment options are limited because resources are limited, for instance, when the preferred treatment option is the most expensive, least available (or unavailable) and/or least proven. A typical case here might be a patient in need of a liver transplantation. If a transplant is definitely not to be made available, there is no justification for continuing with intensive care because it will ultimately give no benefit. Without the liver the patient cannot survive, no matter how aggressive ICU treatment becomes. To continue would be both futile and an inappropriate use of resources. A slightly different case is that of a patient with a very low haemoglobin level who is refusing blood (for instance, a Jehovah's Witness). Once the haemoglobin reaches a critical level for the individual patient ICU treatment loses its therapeutic benefit. There is, however, an alternative. Hyperbaric oxygen therapy has been used in a small number of such patients to increase circulating oxygen during the period when the red blood cells are regenerating[17,18]. Hyperbaric oxygen therapy itself is relatively costly and not widely available, but the real financial cost is borne by the ICU because the patient will remain there for the duration of this and other treatments, often for at least 3–4 weeks. The treatment, though frequently successful, raises a number of concerns, many of which are beyond the scope of this chapter. The issue of most relevance here is that of the justification for expenditure. Should this expensive option be available when the alternative is death or severe brain damage? The issue is additionally clouded by the fact that, in part, the patient's predicament is brought about by his/her refusal of (the much cheaper) conventional therapy. One answer is to return to the consideration of benefits and harms, and whether this consideration should be limited to the individual patient or expanded to cover future ICU patients. Health economists would be able to calculate the real cost of these two options, but suppose that the total cost of treating one patient with hyperbaric oxygen would be enough to treat ten other 'standard' ICU patients. Applying the principle of using resources to maximise benefit, it would be difficult to justify using this therapy because to do so denies future patients a standard option that would otherwise be available. On the other hand, *any* new innovation deviates from what might be given as standard and, if it also happens to be more expensive, it too will come at the price of not being able to treat other patients in the previously standard way. The difficulty with this case is not simply that of how properly to define 'benefit' and 'maximum benefit' but also the role that is played by the patient's own choices. Although maximising benefit is part of what we understand justice to mean, so too is desert, which, in some interpretations, is closely related to individual responsibility.

One legitimate reason to limit intervention is the presence of a patient's advanced directive. Increasingly, patients are limiting their own treatment options in favour of a peaceful death. Provided that the advanced directive is accurate proof of informed choice of a competent patient, it should be upheld as an expression of their autonomy. Advanced directives may influence intervention in at least two ways in an ICU. First, a patient may have made an advanced directive refusing any kind of ICU treatment: not wanting to be admitted to ICU at all. If this is made known prior to admission, then the patient should not be admitted. Second, the advanced directive may express a refusal of consent for certain ICU interventions, such as renal dialysis. In both cases, the instruction is patient initiated, and it may not reflect the patient's views on resource allocation. It could, however, be argued that patients should be encouraged to think, in advance, about what kinds of interventions they would want if they were to become critically ill. If the principle to be applied in resource allocation is that of maximising benefit, then it is important to know what the patient thinks would *not* be of benefit to him or her. In such circumstances, the resource not wanted by one patient can then be used to bring benefit to another patient.

The implementation of advance directives is not without its own difficulties. However, harder still are those cases where a patient or their family is requesting/demanding treatment that the clinician believes offers little or no benefit. Is the clinician legally obliged to give the treatment if the patient or their family demands it? Two legal cases offer precedent on this matter. In *R* v. *Cambridge Health Authority*[19] it was held that the Health Authority had an obligation to take into account service provision as well as individual patients' needs. In the case of *A National Health Service Trust* v. *D and Others*[20], a mother was asking that her child be admitted into an ICU should the need arise, in the face of opposition from the intensivists who thought that the child would not benefit from readmission. The clinical decision was upheld. These legal rulings make it clear that the decision to treat a patient is a clinical one, based on an evaluation of benefits and harms, and it occurs within the context of providing treatment to many patients.

Wenstone suggests that in his experience some relatives welcome decisions to limit ICU treatment based on considerations of resource allocation. Whilst this may be the case for some relatives, others may not be aware of the need for intensivists to consider resource allocation along with other clinical calculations of benefits and harms. In my own experience, relatives often have unrealistic expectations of what ICU treatment can offer and how it affects patients, and they are more likely to be aware of the benefits than the harms. The benefits of ICU are somewhat glamorised by media portrayals but the harms/risks are rarely discussed. When a relative asks for 'everything to be done' they are usually unaware of what effect some treatments have on their loved ones. It would be more beneficial to educate the public, along with colleagues, about the true nature and cost (in all senses) of intensive care, so that users can appreciate that difficult decisions have to be made by clinicians and that some of these decisions need to consider allocation of resources.

Conclusion

Resource allocation is a difficult area of ICU provision but one that is becoming more prominent as clinicians have budget-holding responsibilities. Clinicians are required to account for how they spend the available budget, and they need an equitable system to justify the decisions they make. A consequentialist approach makes an assessment of outcome based on likely benefits and harms, and allows intensivists to consider not only the individual patient but also the future ICU patient population. Using such a system will restrict access to, and some interventions once in, an ICU for some patients if they are assessed as being very unlikely to benefit or very likely to be harmed. It has been argued that the most important aspect of decisions concerning resource allocation is the consistent application of the principle of maximising benefit. Once the ICU team has identified a system that allows clinical judgements to be made in line with Trust policy, applying this system consistently is arguably the most ethical way to be fair. It has further been argued that there is a need for any system to be clear and open, and to be communicated to the public to enable them to understand that decisions are sometimes made with regards to limited resources.

References

1. Department of Health. Guidelines on admission to and discharge from Intensive Care and High Dependency Units. London: HMSO, 1996
2. Department of Health. Comprehensive Critical Care. Review of adult critical care services. London: HMSO, 2001 [http://www.doh.gov.uk/nhsexec/compcritcare.htm]
3. Knaus WA, Draper EA, Wagner DP, Zimmerman JE. APACHE II: a severity of disease scoring classification system. Crit Care Med 1985; 13: 818–29
4. Rubenfeld GD, Crawford SW. Withdrawing life support from mechanically ventilated recipients of bone marrow transplants: a case for evidence-based guidelines. Ann Int Med 1996; 125: 625–33
5. Schönhofer B, Euteneuer S, Nava S, Suchi S, Köhler D. Survival of mechanically ventilated patients admitted to a specialised weaning centre. Intens Care Med 2002; 28: 908–16
6. Heyland DK, Guyatt G, Cook DJ, et al. Frequency and methodologic rigor of quality-of-life assessments in the critical care literature. Crit Care Med 1998; 26: 591–8
7. Vincent JL. European attitudes towards ethical problems in intensive care medicine: results of an ethical questionnaire. Intens Care Med 1990; 16: 256–64
8. Miranda DR, de Rijk A, Schaufeli W. Simplified Therapeutic Intervention Scoring System: The TISS-28 items – Results from a multicenter study. Crit Care Med 1996; 24: 64–73
9. Blanc P, von Elm BE, Geissler A, et al. Economic impact of a rational use of antibiotics in intensive care. Intens Care Med 1999; 25: 1407–12
10. Intensive Care Society. Guidelines for the Transport of the Critically Ill Adult. London: Intensive Care Society (UK), 2002
11. Goldfrad C, Rowan K. Consequences of discharges from intensive care at night. Lancet 2000; 355: 1138–42
12. Daly K, Beale R, Chang RWS. Reduction in mortality after inappropriate early discharge from intensive care unit: logistic regression triage model. Br Med J 2000; 322: 1274–6
13. Audit Commission. Critical to Success: The place of efficient and effective critical care services within the acute hospital. The Audit Commission, 1999

14. Nord E. Cost-Value Analysis in Health Care: Making Sense Out of QALYs. Cambridge: Cambridge University Press, 1999
15. *Bolam* v. *Friern Hospital Management Committee* [1957] 2 All ER 118, [1957] 1 WLR 582
16. *Bolitho* v. *City and Hackney Health Authority* [1997] 39 BMLR 1
17. Bell M. The use of hyperbaric oxygen in the management of severe anaemia in a Jehovahs Witness. Anaesthesia 2000; 55: 293–4
18. McLoughlin PL, Cope TM, Harrison JC. Hyperbaric oxygen therapy in the management of severe acute anaemia in a Jehovahs witness. Anaesthesia 1999; 54: 891–5
19. *R* v. *Cambridge Health Authority* [1995] 1 WLR 898
20. *A National Health Service Trust* v. *D and Others*. The Times, 19 July 2000

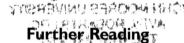

Further Reading

Bion J. Rationing intensive care. Br Med J 1995; 310: 682–3
Scheinkestel CD. The evolution of the intensivist: from health care provider to economic rationalist and ethicist. Med J Austral 1996; 164, 310–12
Skowronski GA. Bed rationing and allocation in the intensive care unit. Curr Opin Crit Care 2001; 7: 480–4
ATS Bioethics Task Force. Fair Allocation of Intensive Care Unit Resources. Am J Resp Crit Care Med 1997; 156, 1282–1301

The Nature of Dilemmas in Intensive Care   12

June Jones

LIVERPOOL
JOHN MOORES UNIVERSITY
AVRIL ROBARTS LRC
TEL. 0151 231 4022

The intensive care unit (ICU) is often a stressful environment in which to work. Many of the illnesses encountered within this specialty expose staff to uncertain prognosis, distressed relatives and increasing pressure to allocate scarce resources equitably. This chapter examines the fundamental nature of dilemmas encountered in an ICU against this background. There is often an underlying assumption about ethics that, because there are no right or wrong answers, there is no way to resolve dilemmas quickly and satisfactorily. In this chapter, it will be argued that, irrespective of whether ethics is capable of providing right and wrong answers, the true nature of some of the dilemmas in intensive care are not identified quickly enough. If they were, there would be more opportunity to resolve the situation to the satisfaction of the multidisciplinary team. This is because, or so it will be argued here, some dilemmas are less to do with ethics per se and more to do with conflicting clinical opinions, the nature of multidisciplinary teamwork and poor communication skills between team members. By reserving the term 'ethical dilemma' for dilemmas that are truly ethical in origin, ICU staff may find that they are able to work together to find an appropriate way forward without so much of the tension that can accompany other types of dilemmas in ICU. Conflicts occurring between professionals and relatives will not be dealt with in this chapter, as there is a wealth of literature already available on this subject[1].

Team decision-making

The need for teamwork in an ICU is obvious. The efforts of no one individual can account for all the complexities of therapy provided for the ICU patient. One aspect of teamwork that has attracted professional attention is that of communication. The Royal College of Anaesthetists (RCOA) guidelines, for instance, suggest:

> Good communications within the directorate are essential if it is to run efficiently and if staff are to feel involved in the department and content in their work. Misunderstandings easily arise and inaccurate perceptions quickly take root. Informal discussions, regular, minuted meetings, letters, memoranda and notice boards form an essential communications network. (p. 11)[2]

Ensuring that all staff involved in patient care are involved with the communication process is an essential aspect of ICU care. Many units have adopted the recommendations within these guidelines by incorporating meetings, notice boards and other such suggestions into the management of ICUs. However, being 'involved in communication' and 'team decision making' are two different things. Being involved in communication may only mean that staff are kept informed of what is going on, whereas team decision making means ensuring that each member of the team is given an opportunity to express his or her considered opinion, in the knowledge that this opinion will be afforded due respect. In the absence of any understanding of what team decision making involves, the process can create tensions between team members.

The most recent British Medical Association (BMA) guidelines on withholding and withdrawing treatment discuss the importance of reaching a consensus in team decision making. Lack of consensus, they claim, 'frequently results from poor communication and inadequate provision of accurate information to all those involved in the decision' (p. 56)[3]. They further recommend that hospital managers put in place conflict management strategies, such as external mediators, to deal with conflicts within the team, and that further independent opinion should be sought if a conflict remains unresolved.

There are several predictable problems that are likely to arise if these guidelines on consensus decision making are implemented. First, there is no notion of lead responsibility. Whilst agreement within the team is desirable, there is no legal requirement for this to occur. On the contrary, it is the admitting consultant and the ICU consultant who have legal responsibility for decision-making. Second, it is clear later in the guidelines that the BMA expect junior doctors and nurses to be involved in the consensus decision making, because it recommends that they be able to 'express informally any misgivings they have about the basis of the decision made' (p. 56)[3]. However, this does not address the fact that junior doctors and nurses have less authority in team decision-making. Recommendations such as these often have two effects. First, they lead to an increased expectation that nurses and junior doctors will be more involved in decision making, but their expectation is often disappointed when they realise how little authority they have in this process. Second, there may be an increased reluctance on behalf of some consultants to act on decisions that do not have the support of their team colleagues.

If consensus is taken to mean a 'general agreement in opinion', then there is an obligation on senior doctors to ask for relevant opinions and to use these to formulate a decision that has support from all concerned. However, in cases where there are conflicting clinical opinions, it is not clear how a consensus can be reached. In decisions concerning the withholding or withdrawal of treatment, a number of aspects of decision making may be involved. Evidence based medicine can be used to facilitate decision making, but this rarely influences decisions about withdrawing care, partly because there is so little relevant evidence available. Previous clinical experience can also be used, but this varies widely, and, if used to inform current decision making, it can be the cause of disagreement amongst team members who may have different experiences. If team members base their decision on their own personal beliefs, team discussion is necessary to ensure that these beliefs can also be supported by clinical and other relevant data concerning the patient to avoid undue personal bias. It is vital, therefore, that team members recognise their obligations to each other, not just to give an opinion but also to discuss how they have reached their opinion, and to take account of the effect that their opinion and instructions may have on other members, which will be discussed later.

The notion of 'patient advocacy' can also result in tensions. Each member of the multidisciplinary team may believe that he or she is responsible for representing the best interests of the patient, whilst each may have a different understanding of how these interests are best served. There is clearly the need in such cases for a lead decision maker who will take overall responsibility for making a decision. This should be the consultant, for the following reasons. Within the team there is no equality of liability: senior clinicians have greatest liability and, therefore, responsibility for the care of the patient. It is because they have the final responsibility that they must also make the final decision. It would be unfair to hold them responsible for decisions over which they did not have total control. It is unlikely that other members of the team would want the immense responsibility that accompanies being the person legally accountable for the decision. This leaves the consultant, however, in the difficult position of both trying to involve everyone but apparently autocratically making the final decision, which may seem to others like the apparent 'team decision' is a fruitless exercise for the sake of appearance. So, consultants need to consider how best to approach their role as lead decision maker.

One approach is to make it clear from the start of the team consultation that the decision is the consultant's to make. It will be easier for the consultant to set the agenda in this way if it is the consultant that initiates the discussion. Tension is often created when junior members of the team feel that senior members are unaware that there is a problem: for instance, the sense amongst some of the team that a patient is no longer benefiting from intervention and, therefore, proceeding is making them feel uncomfortable. If junior members have difficulty bringing such a problem to a consultant's attention because he or she refuses to see it as such, then the consultant's authority to deal with the problem is somewhat eroded. If a consultant initiates the discussion, it is far easier to exercise the authority required. One approach would be for the consultant to ask for opinions to help him or her make the decision. This approach has several benefits. First, this is a statement of the correct legal position, because legally it is the consultant's decision, and he or she will have to take responsibility for it. Second, it indicates that the opinions of other members of the team are being sought, and that their opinions are considered valuable. Most consultants genuinely do value the opinions of other team members, but discussions often occur too late to demonstrate this, leaving juniors with the impression that statements about the value of their opinion is mere rhetoric. Third, discussion of an open-ended, clearly stated problem tends to be less adversarial (and, therefore, more likely to yield relevant information) than a discussion to defend a decision that already seems to have been made.

165

Professional relationships and responsibilities

The effectiveness of communication and teamwork directly affect professional relationships within the multidisciplinary ICU team. The RCOA guidelines acknowledge the importance of maintaining good professional relationships, the lead role anaesthetists often play in decision making and the need for 'robust debate' in the professional practice of this role.

> The ability to work harmoniously in departments and teams is essential if patients are to be cared for properly. Anaesthetists will often take a lead in decision-making and robust debate within departments and with other groups is an essential component in providing high quality anaesthetic service. However, there is no place in modern anaesthetic departments for individuals who pursue their clinical practice and style of personal conduct irrespective of the views and wishes of their colleagues. Professional independence is important and variety is healthy, both in clinical practice and personal style, but the limits of acceptable behaviour must be recognised by all concerned. (p. 9)[2]

The RCOA clearly recognises a difference between acceptable and unacceptable behaviour but, in common with other similar guidelines, does not say how to distinguish between them. This places other colleagues in a difficult position.

How is one to judge if another colleague is behaving in an unacceptable manner during the decision-making process? Beckerman *et al.* argue that one type of unacceptable behaviour is failure to protect colleagues from needless harm. He wants to extend the concept of non-maleficence, normally used to discuss duties towards patients, to the treatment of our colleagues within the multidisciplinary team.

> Is the right to protection from needless harm limited to patients? Is there a parallel need for physicians to avoid needless harm to themselves or to each other in the course of their work as individuals and members of a team? . . . If physicians have an obligation not to harm patients, it is reasonable to assume that they also have an obligation to treat each other in ways that enable themselves and others to sustain and even enhance their capacity for caring for patients . . . there is a significant relationship between care of staff and care of patients. (pp. 35–7)[4]

This is an interesting argument because the duty owed to colleagues not to cause harm is extended beyond physical harm (for instance, avoiding causing needle-stick injuries to colleagues) to that of psychological harm (for instance, lack of discussion/involvement in decision making). This initially appears a weak position to defend because it seems to employ too wide a notion of the duty of non-maleficence. Too wide a duty to avoid harming others may become impractical – for example, if we include harm that is difficult to foresee, as is often the case with psychological harm. However, this argument would be more defensible if it could be shown that this type of harm is predictable and that it could be avoided by being involved in the decision-making process.

Inter-professional disagreements

The BMA recognise that nurses are adversely affected by not being involved in decisions concerning the patients in their care, and they suffer further adverse affects when they are required to implement the decisions with which they disagree.

> The importance of team working in providing health care is widely recognised and is particularly important when making complex decisions about whether to withhold or withdraw life-prolonging treatment . . . All health professionals involved with caring for the patient have an important contribution to make to the assessment; nurses often have a particular insight . . . many nurses have reported concerns about what they perceive as the 'moral distancing' on the part of some doctors. They consider that those who make the decisions generally delegate its implementation to nurses, who can feel unhappy if they have not been able to contribute in any way to that decision. (p. 53)[3]

The BMA acknowledge that nurses and junior doctors are sometimes left in a position where they have to carry out treatments that they believe are morally wrong, without having the opportunity to raise their concerns. Involving nurses and junior doctors in the decision-making process does not, however, guarantee that their views will prevail. Accordingly, they may still be required to give treatments they believe to be morally wrong if a decision with which they disagree is made.

Should any health-care professional be required to carry out instructions they believe to be morally wrong? The Nuremberg trials demonstrated that carrying out orders is no defence, but the nature of those orders, the penalty for not complying and the resulting violation of human rights makes this comparison unhelpful within a health-care context. An example from Beckerman *et al.*[4] illustrates a type of dilemma likely to be encountered by ICU staff:

An elderly lady with a terminal illness was admitted to the ICU for mechanical ventilation and cardiac support. The junior doctors interpreted her agitation as evidence of pain, requiring sedation. The admitting consultant believed that sedating the patient would cause her death and so would not allow sedation to be given. A subsequent review of her case noted that there was an

> . . . explicit acknowledgement that to sedate or not to sedate was more likely to be determined by medical seniority than by expert medical knowledge. Medical decisions are often made in a hierarchical structure, with the understanding – but not necessarily agreement – among the junior team members. (p. 35)[4]

The members of the team implementing that decision felt they were harming the patient by performing invasive procedures, such as endotracheal suctioning, without sedation. The invasive nature of ICU therapy tends to distress patients who are not sedated and, because junior team members believed she was in pain, it is conceivable that *they too* were actually harmed by being required to give care that they perceived to be contributing to her distress. There can be no obligation to perform tasks that one strongly disagrees with. Senior doctors must not only be willing to give instructions, but also be prepared to administer them if junior colleagues refuse. Such occasions where this would be necessary should be rare, but they may be avoidable altogether if good communication and team decision making were employed.

Obviously, treatment plans cannot be dictated solely by whether team members perceive themselves to be harmed by the care they are instructed to give; decisions have to be based in the best interest of the patient, not the staff. However, sometimes this might just be a matter of perception. In this case, there was a conflict over which of the two ethical principles of beneficence and non-maleficence was the most important. The junior doctors believed that sedation was in the patient's best interest (beneficence) but the senior doctor believed that he had a duty not to harm the patient by killing her (non-maleficence), and believed that her death was an avoidable harm. Discussion around clinical data was needed to address these two conflicting views. The junior doctors may have revised their position if it could have been demonstrated that treatment without sedation was, in fact, not harmful. This may have been achieved by showing that their perception of the patient's pain and distress was false, or by showing that their perception was accurate and raising the possibility that she could have been given an analgesia that did not cause sedation. Alternatively, it may have been possible to alter the perception of the senior doctor, perhaps by showing that sedation would not have led to the patient's death, or by arguing that sedating this patient, even if she did die, would not have been a harm. It may even have been possible to discuss whether her death would have been directly caused by the sedation, or whether the true cause of the death would have been the disease process. Either way, if the clinical facts could have been ascertained, no ethical dilemma would have existed because the facts would have told either in favour of sedation or not.

In deciding to withhold sedation, the senior doctor required the junior staff to give treatments they morally disagreed with. In this case, all members of the team needed to discuss the treatment plan, and full rationale needed to be provided, no matter what time of day or night the case occurred. If the junior staff remained unwilling to treat without sedation, the senior doctor should have attended and delivered the treatment personally until the conflict was resolved. To expect junior colleagues to carry out requests with which they disagree is unacceptable because the treatment plan was non-standard and there had been no prior consultation of non-standard treatment plans. This type of problem needs to be resolved as a matter of urgency whenever it arises.

The decision to treat someone invasively without sedation is a clinical decision, made on clinical grounds. The grounds are usually that to use sedation would compromise respiratory function to a critical level. The reason for not wanting to compromise respiratory function with sedation would commonly be that there is genuine concern about the inability to wean the patient off a ventilator once that treatment is commenced. This is a clinical, not ethical decision. It obviously has ethical overtones, and ethical language might be used to discuss the case, but a purely ethical debate would miss the point. The consultant has to justify whether starting sedation would (a) cause the patient's death or (b) render the patient so dependent on equipment to maintain life that they could not justify commencing it. This is a different scenario to the majority of cases where a patient is critically ill and needs life support. In these cases, treatment is commenced with the expectation of successful weaning. Exceptionally, however, there are patients where it can be predicted that treatment would make them dependent on ventilation for the rest of their lives. This being the case, sedation would be wrong because it would start the cascade of treatment that could not be justified by the long-term outcome. These concerns do not appear to have been present in this case because ventilation was started, but was administered without sedation. This led to care being given to a distressed and terminally ill patient by traumatised staff for reasons that appeared unacceptable to them.

A case that demonstrates how another type of dilemma was resolved is the famous American Wanglie case[5]. Mrs Wanglie was in permanent vegetative state (PVS), and her multidisciplinary team judged therapy to be inappropriate but her family insisted on it being continued. The focus of the clinical case concerned the conflict between the health-care practitioners and the family, and the resulting court case, but Miles draws attention to factors that affected the teamwork of the health-care practioners, especially the nurses:

> The nurses were feeling trapped by an endless treatment plan that obliged them to provide treatment they did not believe was appropriate or could benefit a dying patient . . . taking the case to court marked a turning point in the morale of the nurses. Even though Mrs Wanglie's treatment continued for many months, the nurses felt they had been heard; the delayed resolution of the dispute now resulted from legal procedures rather than a patronizing attitude of co-workers. (pp. 62–3)[5]

Miles seems to suggest that the nurses involved in this case were vulnerable: they carried out treatment plans they believe to be wrong, because they felt powerless to withdraw their cooperation. Nurses would rarely take the step of withdrawing cooperation because they disagree with a treatment plan; and, because they have limited authority in these matters, they are often placed in a difficult position between two mutually incompatible sets of duties. Nurses are employed to provide ICU care to patients as part of the multidisciplinary team, and are instructed by their Code of Conduct to 'cooperate with others in the team' (point 4)[6]. However, nurses continue to have legal responsibilities to act in the best interests of their patients. In cases where ICU nurses perceive care to be contrary to the patient's interests, they cannot at the same time fulfil their contractual obligations and their professional obligations. Nurses in ICUs may not be considered a typically vulnerable group because they are often a most vocal group of specialist nurses, but their lack of substantial professional autonomy does create real ethical dilemmas because it can render them powerless to resist the orders of a colleague with greater authority. The solution to this inherent problem lies in multidisciplinary team members recognising the professional boundaries that they each work within.

Another aspect of the Wanglie case was the change brought about by the court case. The tension between team members dissipated when they all perceived themselves to be 'on the same side'. It is regrettable that it took a court case to achieve this when it could have been done by good communication along with a desire to reduce the vulnerability experienced by nurses and junior doctors, who may feel trapped into providing care with which they disagree.

The nature of an ethical dilemma

Ethical dilemmas arise when one situation has two available courses of action and there is genuine uncertainty about which course of action to pursue. Two forms of ethical dilemmas have been identified:

> (a) Some evidence indicates that act x is morally right, and some evidence indicates that act x is morally wrong, but the evidence on both sides is inconclusive . . . (b) An agent believes that, on moral grounds, he or she both ought and ought not to perform act x. In a moral dilemma with this form, an agent is obligated by one or more moral norms to do x and obligated by one or more moral norms to do y, but the agent is precluded in the circumstances from doing both. (p. 11)[7]

In the first form of an ethical dilemma, a proposed action would need to have elements in it that were both morally right and wrong, but the evidence normally used to aid decision making would be unhelpful because it is not decisive. An example of this kind of dilemma can be seen when a patient is taken from ICU for a computed tomography (CT) scan of their abdomen, with the hope of locating the source of sepsis. If the scan is negative, it may be difficult to justify surgery because of the additional associated risks where no primary source has been identified. In this case, there is no clinical certainty with which to plan a course of action. Some evidence (the sepsis) indicates that surgery is morally right and some evidence (the CT scan and the increased risks) indicates that surgery is morally wrong, but the clinical evidence for and against surgery is inconclusive. This type of dilemma tends to be seen as more of a clinical dilemma because the information used to make treatment decisions is primarily based on interpreting clinical data, not ethical data. There is, however, an ethical dimension because the primary duty of the surgeon is to do no harm, but he or she does not have the conclusive evidence upon which to fulfil this obligation.

In the second form, an ethical dilemma arises because performing one morally required action directly contravenes another duty held in equally high regard. Such was the case with Tony Bland. The *Bland* case[8] raised two genuinely conflicting duties: the ethical requirement not to kill versus the ethical duty not to continue with futile therapy. Withdrawing Bland's artificial feeding (the futile therapy) would bring about his death (and would be tantamount to killing him in the eyes of many people). Furthermore, health care professionals are morally obliged to provide feeding for their patients, but, in the case of Bland, continuing to provide feeding was seen as morally wrong because it could not benefit him. The case of Bland generated a genuine ethical dilemma: staff could not both give and withhold artificial feeding. Post-Bland, it is now standard to consider the concept of futility when considering withdrawal of therapy. The concept of futility has changed the nature of the moral obligation because it explains why we are *not* morally obligated to do both *x* and *y* under these particular circumstances.

Futility and ethical dilemmas

The concept of futility seems to be one that has made ethical decision making in ICU both transparent and defensible. However, there is uncertainty as to how futility is to be defined. It may be interpreted as a therapy that cannot produce *any* result and would, therefore, be pointless, or it may be taken to mean a treatment that cannot reverse the decline in a patient. This is an important distinction because most ICU therapies can usually produce some result, no matter how small. This can be demonstrated in biochemical changes, oxygen consumption or urine output. If the former definition were to be adopted as the working definition of futility, the majority of ICU therapy for most patients would have to be continued to the point where no result of any type could be expected from therapy. If, on the other hand, the working definition of futility were to be a therapy that would be unable to reverse the decline of a patient, it would exclude therapies where a small biochemical change was effected with no overall change to the outcome. This may be the preferred definition for intensive care, but it is one that is harder to judge consistently. This is mainly because the concept of futility involves both qualitative and quantitative elements. It is not just skill in clinical judgement that is being called for, but ethical judgements about when a therapy ceases to benefit because it is unable to reverse the decline of the patient. This is because clinicians identify the *irreversible* nature of the decline at differing points. Some clinicians may accept that a patient is generally declining but may also see small improvements as being clinically significant, whilst others may not find encouragement in small improvements, believing that any small 'improvements' will merely provide false hope to relatives if not communicated effectively. Thus, a situation often occurs where some members of the team consider intervention to have become futile before other members are prepared to accept this. The BMA recognises this tension between the uncertain nature of medicine and the perceived need for certainty prior to decision making:

> Despite being evidence based, some aspects of medical treatment will always remain uncertain. Death is a certainty for everyone but, except in a small number of cases, diagnosis and prognosis are based on probability and past experience rather than absolute certainty. (p. 11)[3]

Where there is no therapeutic justification, there can be no moral obligation to continue or to commence such treatment. However futility is defined, once it is agreed that treatment is not in the best interests of the incompetent patient, it loses its therapeutic justification. As Lord Brown, speaking in the Bland judgment, asserted:

171

In my judgement, it must follow from this that if there comes a stage where the responsible doctor comes to the reasonable conclusion (which accords with the views of a responsible body of medical opinion) that further continuance of an intrusive life support system is not in the best interests of the patient, he can no longer lawfully continue that life support system: to do so would constitute the crime of battery and the torte of trespass to the person. Therefore he cannot be in breach of any duty to maintain the patient's life. Therefore he is not guilty of murder by omission. (p. 855)[9]

Where there is no moral obligation, there is no ethical dilemma, although practical dilemmas may remain. These centre around how to move into the palliative phase of care, what, or in what order, interventions should be withdrawn to achieve palliation and how best to communicate the change in emphasis to the relatives effectively. These outstanding practical problems should not be confused with ethical dilemmas, which ceased once the interventions were determined to be futile.

Conclusion

If ICU team members resolve conflicts arising from poor communication, lack of teamwork and lack of understanding of professional roles and responsibilities, what kind of dilemmas should be called ethical ones? This chapter has shown that at least some of the apparently ethical dilemmas in ICU are actually problems that arise from poor inter-professional communication and the absence of clearly defined mechanisms for team decision making. In this respect, although they create ethical problems for ICU staff, the initiating event may not have been one with an ethical dimension at all. This does not mean, however, that there are no ethical dilemmas in intensive care. Ethical dilemmas will arise in ICUs because treatment plans can vary so much; two clinical opinions may be both valid and conflicting. Where the patient is incompetent, the consultants need to discuss both options with the multidisciplinary team and the relatives, and then make a decision based on the best interests of the patient. If there is doubt over the legality of the treatment proposal, a court ruling may be sought. It may, at first sight, appear that there is no right or wrong answer, but when clarity is sought the decision often becomes part of professional consensus guidelines. Prior to *Bland*[8], there was no legal clarity on stopping artificial feeding on patients who had no hope of recovery, but, following *Bland*, professional guidelines were developed, which provide good clinical guidance for ICU clinicians. Ethical dilemmas will also continue because of disagreements between relatives and health-care professionals, with conflict over how best to decide what is in the best interest of the patient. These dilemmas may actually be the real ethical dilemmas in ICUs. The care of a critically ill patient causes many conflicts. Where the conflicts are between team members, good communication, teamwork and professional understanding can often reduce these dilemmas to a minimum, and only when these are achieved can the true nature of ethical dilemmas in ICU really be seen.

References

1. Seymour AE. Critical Moments: Death and Dying in Intensive Care. Buckingham PA: Open University Press, 2001
2. Royal College of Anaesthetists. Good Practice: A Guide for Departments of Anaesthesia. London: Royal College of Anaesthetists, 1998
3. British Medical Association. Withholding and Withdrawing Life-prolonging Medical Treatment: guidance for decision-making. London: British Medical Association Publications, 2001
4. Beckerman A, Doerfler M, Couch E, Lowenstein J. Ethical issues and relationships between house staff and attending physicians: a case study. J Clin Ethics 1997; 8: 34–8
5. Miles SH. Interpersonal issues in the Wanglie case. Kennedy Inst Ethics J 1992; 2: 61–72
6. Nursing and Midwifery Council. Code of Professional Conduct, April 2002. http://www.nmc-uk.org/cms/content/Publications/Code
7. Beauchamps TL, Childress JF. Principles of Biomedical Ethics. 4th edn. Oxford: Oxford University Press, 1994
8. *Airedale NHS Trust* v. *Bland* [1993] 1 All ER 821
9. McHale, Fox Health Care Law. London: Sweet & Maxwell, 1997

Further Reading

Zucker MB, Zucker HD. Medical Futility. Cambridge: Cambridge University Press, 1997
Ravenscroft AJ, Bell DMD. End of life decision making within intensive care – objective, consistent, defensible? J Med Ethics 2000; 26: 435–40
Street K, Ashcroft R, Henderson J, Campbell AV. The decision making process regarding the withdrawal or withholding of potential life-saving treatments in a children's hospital. J Med Ethics 2000; 26: 346–52

Withdrawing and Withholding Life-sustaining Therapy and Euthanasia

13

Heather Draper

Introduction

Kipnis draws a distinction between 'consensus' issues in medical ethics, and 'knife-edge' issues[1]. Consensus issues are those where, whilst there might have been a history of heated debate, a consensus has by and large been reached by the medical profession. Evidence of a consensus is provided when bodies such as the General Medical Council (GMC), British Medical Association (BMA) or Royal Colleges produce guidelines, which, in turn, would be used by the courts in their assessment of reasonable practice, for instance in the application of the Bolam[2] principle*. Knife-edge issues, on the other hand, are those where there is on-going disagreement over what the right or wrong thing to do might be.

There seems to be an emerging consensus about withholding and withdrawing therapy – as evidenced by the guidelines produced by the GMC[3], BMA[4], the judgment in the case of *Bland*[5] and the recent failure of the Private Member's Bill that was designed to require doctors not to withhold or withdraw life-sustaining therapy from any patients, save those who actively and competently refused it. Likewise, one might suppose that, because there are frequent calls for a change in the law prohibiting euthanasia, euthanasia remains a knife-edge issue. In this chapter, I will argue that, whilst there is some consensus on the issue of withdrawing and withholding life-sustaining therapy, this consensus is only skin-deep and it masks many knife-edge issues. Euthanasia, on the other hand, appears to be a knife-edge issue, but I will argue there will be greater potential for consensus once various confusions about what euthanasia is, and is not, are sorted out.

I start by looking at withdrawing and withholding therapy. I will outline some of the areas of apparent consensus that have emerged in UK law since

---

*The Bolam principle is that doctors will not be found to have acted negligently provided that their practice conforms to a reasonable body of medical opinion. It takes its name from the case *Bolam v. Friern Hospital Management Committee*[2].

the *Bland* case[5], and in the ethics of the profession, evidenced by the BMA's and GMC's guidelines on withdrawing and withholding therapy[3,4]. Paying particular attention to the BMA guidelines, I will then show that behind the apparent consensus there lie many unresolved 'knife-edge' issues. Finally, I will look at euthanasia and the distinction between killing and allowing to die, some acts and omissions commonly confused with euthanasia, and, finally, whether clarifying what euthanasia *is* – or perhaps more importantly, *is not* – goes some way to laying the ground for a consensus that reflects the current law.

Withdrawing and withholding life-prolonging therapy: evidence of consensus and outstanding knife-edge issues

Competent refusal of treatment

It is now almost universally agreed that competent patients are entitled to refuse treatment, even that necessary to save their lives[6]. Areas of disagreement tend to centre on whether a patient is actually competent[7] and on Gillick competent children (see Chapter 6). Likewise, there is growing acceptance of living wills that enable competent patients to refuse treatment in advance of becoming incapable of doing so.

In relation to withdrawing and withholding life-sustaining treatment there remain, however, some outstanding grey areas, and even knife-edge issues, that should not be overlooked. One grey area, which will not be discussed at length here, is whether a competent pregnant woman can refuse treatment when to do so will endanger the life of the foetus. Whilst common law in the UK suggests that she may[8,9], a case has yet to be brought under the Human Rights Act (1998), which could be interpreted as affording the same right to life to the foetus as to any other human being.

On the face of it, refusal of consent should be uncontroversial – a competent patient, as Lord Templeman said, has a right to refuse treatment for any reason, no reason, or even irrational reasons[10]. As the following series of questions illustrates, however, cases can arise that might not be this straightforward.

Can respecting a refusal of consent be tantamount to assisting a self-killing?

Both euthanasia and assisted self-killing are illegal in the UK, and the law draws no distinction between active and passive euthanasia. Elsewhere, I have argued that a competent refusal of life-sustaining treatment should not be confused with euthanasia, even when the patient is using the refusal as a means of bringing about his or her own death in circumstances akin to those associated with passive euthanasia[7]. A similar argument could be made, however, in relation to assisted self-killing. Montgomery, for instance, suggests that a distinction could be drawn between what a patient does for themselves (i.e. physically turning off their own life-support machine) and what the patient asks someone else to do because they are incapable of acting upon their own desires (i.e. asking someone else to turn off the life-support machine)[11].* The argument implied by this distinction runs like this: if it is wrong actively to help someone to kill themselves, even when they are incapable of doing so alone, it must also be wrong to help someone kill themselves by omission, or passively, even if they are incapable of doing this alone. The grey area that now emerges is whether the reason given by the patient for refusing life-sustaining treatment affects the rights or wrongs of complying with their wishes.

In their guidelines on refusal of consent, the BMA focuses on the sort of patient who decides that the burdens of the therapy are no longer outweighed by its benefits, even when the benefit is the chance of a longer life. It is clear that they are assuming that both the doctor and the patient are making the same kind of judgement, namely one about the potential to benefit from the *treatment*. However, this may not be the case at all. Rather than making a judgement about the benefits and burdens of treatment, the patient may be actively seeking death (by one means or another, or by the easiest means, or perhaps even by the only means he or she feels is available). From the patient's point of view, acceding to this request is aiding self-killing, whereas from the doctor's point of view, a failure to comply with a refusal of treatment is battery. Kennedy resolves this problem by arguing that in turning off the life-support machine the doctor simply enables the patient to choose either to have it turned on again or to choose death[12]. This is a rather ingenious interpretation. A more straightforward argument is that it is acceptable to separate what the patient intends from what the doctor intends. The doctor is obliged not to give treatment without the consent of the patient. Accordingly, if a competent patient refuses treatment then the doctor has no choice but to comply and withdraw the treatment: the doctor's intention is to avoid a battery even if the patient's intention is to bring about their own death. The doctor and the patient have to be judged according to their own, rather than each other's, intentions. The potential moral objection here centres not on what the doctor does but on what the patient does, since the patient is using the doctor as a means to the end of achieving the slightly different agenda of dying. If, however, the doctor agrees with the patient's intentions – consents to enable the patient to die – then the doctor would be responsible for assisting a self-killing.

Is there a potential gender bias in competent refusal of life-sustaining therapy? Biggs identifies another grey area in competent decision-making: the possibility of gender bias[13]. In the case of refusal of life-sustaining treatment she draws our attention to the fact that women are often the primary carers of the sick. They are, therefore, in the best position to know what a burden providing long-term care can be.

> (M)any women's perceptions and tolerance of their own illnesses and infirmities are inescapably coloured by their own experience as carers. They know what is involved because they have been responsible for doing it, or have at least supported others who have done it. (p. 292)[13]

---

*Montgomery discusses this example as being equivalent to voluntary euthanasia – but he confused assisted self-killing with euthanasia.

Accordingly, she argues that women are likely to be reluctant to place this burden upon others. Biggs is aware that her work has two very different implications. The first is that women feel more vulnerable as patients, and more concerned about the effects that their decisions to continue with life-sustaining treatment might have on others. Doctors may need, therefore, to take particular care to ensure that women who fall into this category are not placing undue weight on the effect that their illness is having on others, but instead are reassured that they should make decisions based on what they personally want. The second implication is that women are actually making a more considered response to treatment decisions, and that they are more willing to take responsibility for the consequences of their decisions on other people. Under this interpretation, women might be more informed decision makers than men.

What limits should be placed on competent patients' decisions?   How much control over life-sustaining therapies can a competent patient be afforded? We are now moving from grey areas into more controversial issues. The BMA distinguishes between a patient refusing treatment and a patient insisting upon treatment. They argue that patients' rights are limited to a refusal of therapy and do not extend to insisting either on treatment per se or any particular treatment (p. 20)[4]. This is a position echoed by the GMC (p. 10)[3]. In the opinion of the BMA, this includes not only cases where the treatment 'cannot produce the desired benefit' (p. 21)[4] but also those cases where treatment would be 'contrary to an individual's health interests' because it will 'result in severe pain or loss of function' *despite the fact* that it will 'prolong life' (p. 22)[4]. Whilst I agree that patients should not get what they want simply because they want it[14], what the BMA is suggesting here needs some careful reflection.

  In the discussion that accompanies the guidance related to treatment that 'cannot produce the desired benefit', the BMA accept that treatment that has little long-term benefit may be given to help a patient achieve a particular goal (they do not give examples here, but one could suppose that these would include the surviving long enough to witness the birth of a grandchild, attend a child's wedding, or to give birth to one's own child). Resource implications aside, this seem fairly uncontentious. There is, however, a tension between acknowledging, on the one hand, that 'the patient's own view about the acceptable level of burden or risk . . . will carry weight in assessing the overall benefit of the treatment to the patient . . . (such that) . . . if the patient knows and has accepted the chance and level of expected recovery and wishes to accept treatment on that basis it would be difficult to say that this treatment is of no benefit to that patient' (p. 21)[4], and, on the other hand, to assert that doctors are 'not obliged to provide treatment contrary to their clinical judgement' (p. 22)[4]. The tension exists because it is not obvious that the clinical judgement should *necessarily* be informed by what the patient believes on balance to be the case.

  The BMA guidance specifically refers to treatment requested by the patient that is contrary to their 'health interests'. Presumably the reference to the patient's interests is prefixed by 'health' to distinguish this health-related interest from other interests, such as those related to the patient's autonomy. This suggests that, if the patient cannot ultimately be persuaded to agree with the clinical judgement, it is acceptable for the doctor simply to do what he or she thinks is best, regardless of the patient's judgement. Or perhaps this could be put another way: once the doctor has decided that the treatment will not benefit the patient, the patient must be given the opportunity to dissuade them, but, if that fails, the doctor may do what he or she judges to be best. This might be reasonable when the patient is articulate, but it may not be sufficient to ensure that the less articulate are able to influence the balance that has to be drawn between health interests and other interests.

But there is an additional implication for consent here. Elsewhere in their guidance, the BMA recommends that the patient should be given 'information about the treatment proposed, the consequences of not having the treatment and any alternative forms of treatment available' (p. 16)[4]. If the two pieces of advice are taken together, the 'proposed' treatment and the 'alternative' treatments referred to must mean those that the doctor is actually prepared to give, as opposed to those that are actually available. Yet, there is a strong relationship between information giving and coercion. If the information is tailored to suit the outcome that the doctor deems acceptable then the patient's consent is not fully voluntary, as he or she may have decided otherwise if they had been given information about treatments that the doctor was not prepared to give. They may, for instance, have decided to ask for a second opinion, or to be transferred to a doctor who was prepared to offer these treatments, perhaps attending as a private patient if necessary.

As it happens, I actually agree with the BMA that the reasonable and competent clinician should have the ultimate say in what treatment is given. This is because it is the doctor who is ultimately legally responsible for what is done, but this message is not spelt out the guidance. Why? There are at least two potential explanations. The first is that the BMA is focusing on good practice. Where there is a good relationship between doctor and patient, there is greater scope for mutually agreed decisions that treatment should be withdrawn, or no further active treatment options pursued. A second explanation is that the profession is reluctant to assert its rights against patients in the prevailing climate of deference to patient autonomy. Either way, it would not be surprising if patients' rights organisations take exception to doctors tailoring information to suit what they themselves want to achieve, rather than allowing their patients to decide what is appropriate for them.

Must patients exhibit a greater level of competence when they refuse treatment? Another controversy relates to the practice of overriding a patient's refusal of consent to life-sustaining therapy by claiming that they are actually incompetent (usually *because* they have refused therapy). This enables the practitioner to follow their own desired course of action in the patient's best interests (because once a patient is considered to be incompetent, the practitioner has a duty to decide on this basis).

Discussion of this kind of practice can move in one of two directions. The first is a philosophical debate about whether greater competence is required to act against expert advice than to agree with expert advice: this debate will be outlined shortly. The second direction is that the practice typifies the balance that has to be struck between autonomy on the one hand and beneficence on the other, and this is an area of significant controversy in academic medical ethics.

For some writers, there is no tension between beneficence and autonomy because the least beneficent thing one can do to a person is to override their autonomy. The balance, if that is indeed the appropriate terminology from this perspective, therefore, always swings in favour of autonomy. Other commentators point out that this kind of analysis overlooks the autonomy of the practitioner. Practitioners are not mere technicians for hire; they are also moral agents in their own right, who are responsible for their actions, and must, therefore, only do what they believe to be right. Now, there are examples of bad practice on both sides here, and both sides must acknowledge this. Some patients are capable of making very unreasonable demands on the basis that they have certain rights over their own bodies or over their own medical treatment. Equally, some practitioners can show an arrogant disregard for their patients whose sole purpose seems to be that they are the means to the end of practising medicine. There lie, in between these extremes, many cases of reasonable and genuine disagreement between doctor and patient over the best course of action. An apparent consensus on respect for a competent refusal of consent should not be permitted to mask a knife-edge issue, such as how best to tackle the issue of competing views about best interests.

The philosophical debate about competence is no less difficult. The practice of declaring patients incompetent once they reject medical advice seems to go against the fourth element of consent, which suggests that once a patient has made a decision, it should be respected whatever that decision turns out to be. It seems obvious that if the patient was competent to decide to follow medical advice, then they were equally competent to disregard that advice. But is this assumption justified? Arguably not, because the decision to act against expert advice is more complex and risky than the decision to follow expert advice[15,16]. Since the assessment of a patient's competence is related to the complexity of the decision to be made, it then seems reasonable to suppose that a patient must be more competent to reject medical advice than to accept it. This is precisely the line of reasoning that is used to justify overriding the refusal of consent of a Gillick competent child when their consent would have been sufficient to permit the treatment to go ahead.

Conclusion   The refusal of a competent patient to accept life-sustaining treatment should be the least controversial topic for discussion. As the above questions show, however, even here lurk knife-edge issues that can threaten apparent consensus. These difficult issues cannot be ignored if the consensus is to continue, for they may lie at the heart of some of the tensions between practitioners that are discussed in Chapter 12.

Airedale NHS Trust v. Bland

The judgement by the House of Lords in the case referred to simply as *Bland*[5] has become *the* yardstick against which other cases of withholding/withdrawing treatment are measured. This has happened despite the warning by the Lords that the judgment in *Bland* should not be viewed as a precedent case. In *French NHS Trust* v. *S*[17], it was suggested that cases involving patients in a permanent vegetative state (PVS) need not even come to court – though a Practice Note from the Official Solicitor suggests otherwise[18]. The facts in *Bland* are widely known.* What is important for the purposes of this chapter is to outline the principles that *Bland* has established for the withdrawing, or withholding, of life-sustaining therapies.

Although *Bland* should, strictly speaking, only apply to patients in PVS, several general principles emerged that have been used more broadly in cases where life-sustaining treatment is to be withdrawn. First, there is absolutely no obligation on doctors to maintain life; rather, all treatment (and in *Bland* it was also established that artificial feeding constituted a therapy) should be given or withheld with reference to the doctor's assessment of the patient's best interests, which in turn could be tested against *Bolam*[2] in cases of dispute.† Indeed, rather than arguing that the failure to maintain life should always be regarded as a homicide, Lord Brown-Wilkinson argued that it would actually be unlawful for a doctor to continue with life-sustaining therapy that he or she believed was not in the patient's best interests.

A second important principle established in *Bland* was that no distinction should be drawn between withdrawing and withholding treatment. As Lord Lowery said, any decision to the contrary would 'quite illogically confer on a doctor who had refrained from treatment an immunity which did not benefit a doctor who had embarked on treatment in order to see whether it might benefit the patient and had abandoned . . . (it) . . . when it was seen not to do so.'[5] Clearly, then, it is not in the interests of the public that a doctor feels unable to seize the chance of life for a patient because the doctor is afraid that so doing might commit them to protracting the dying process against the patient's interests.

The *Bland* judgment has withstood the introduction of the Human Rights Act (1998), Article 2 of which asserts a universal human right to life. Article 3, on the other hand, is thought to support *Bland* because it demands protection from 'inhuman or degrading treatment'. Doctors, as public agents, are obliged to give both articles due weight. However, Article 2, whilst suggesting a positive duty, is not taken to imply that everything possible must be done to save life, and Article 3 is likely to carry greater weight in those cases where patients themselves

---

*Tony Bland was one of the spectators who were crushed in the Hillsborough Stadium disaster. Although he survived, he was left in a permanent vegetative state and his doctors sought permission from the coroner to stop tube-feeding him. Bland's parents supported the action of the doctors. The coroner warned the doctors that he could not condone such an action as the law stood, so the case was passed to the courts to determine what was in the best interests of Bland (as an incompetent adult, for whom no legal proxy consent could be given). The case went all the way to the House of Lords, who decided that the doctors could withdraw artificial feeding in the case. Bland died several weeks later.

†Though if a case did come to court, it would then be the court that determined whether the doctor's behaviour was reasonable – taking all the available evidence into account. The case of *Bolitho* v. *Hackney HA* [1993] 4 Med. LR 381 has made clear that the court does not have to simply acquiesce to the profession's interpretation of reasonable behaviour, but is free to decide whether the behaviour is reasonable in the opinion of the court.

ones in their own. The additional positive weight is supplied by experience itself, rather than by any of its content. (p. 2)[23]

And this view is prominent not only in philosophy but also in Roman Catholicism, Judaism and Islam.

The quality of life compared with the intrinsic value of life is not the only bone of contention. If the quality of life view has primacy, the BMA has to provide some guidance to doctors on how quality of life is to be assessed – particularly in relation to the case-by-case assessment of best interests of incompetent patients. They say: '(w)here . . . the disability is so profound that individuals have no or minimal levels of awareness of their own existence and no hope of recovering awareness, or where they suffer severe untreatable pain or other distress' (p. 4)[4], that it is not obvious that continuing to live can be classed as a benefit. Awareness is defined (p. 4)[4] as:

- being able to interact with others
- being aware of his or her own existence and having the ability to take pleasure in the fact of that existence
- having the ability to achieve some purpose or self-directed action or to achieve some goal of importance to him or herself.

It is not surprising that awareness has such a prominent place in the determination of quality of life. In *Bland*[5], it was argued that Tony Bland had no best interests because he had no interests *at all*, and the reason that he had no interests at all was because he had no mental capacity whatsoever, even sentience was absent. Indeed, it has even been argued that the concept of death should be redefined to take into account cases where brain function has irreversibly fallen below that necessary for self-awareness of any kind[22]. Since another area of undoubted consensus is that treating the dead can be of no benefit to them, it is important for us to agree about what constitutes death, and it is by no means obvious that the time is ripe for a redefinition from the brain-stem criteria to that focusing on lack of consciousness (see Chapter 14).

Returning to the assessment of best interests, the BMA recommend that account should be taken of the following (pp. 52–3)[4]:

- the patient's own wishes and values (where these can be ascertained)
- clinical judgement about the effectiveness of the proposed treatment
- the likelihood of the patient experiencing severe unmanageable pain or suffering
- the level of awareness the individual has of his or her existence and surroundings
- the likelihood and extent of any degree of improvement in the patient's condition if treatment is provided
- whether the invasiveness is justified in the circumstances
- the views of the parents, if the patient is a child
- the views of people close to the patient, especially close relatives, partners and carers, about what the patient is likely to see as beneficial
- in Scotland; the views of an appointed health-care proxy.

There is the danger of a circular argument beginning to emerge here as the benefit of the treatment is defined partly in term of quality of life, and quality of life is partly determined by the capacity of the patient to benefit from treatment.

Separating the value of the treatment from the value of the patient.   In order to avoid another area of contention – namely, that which claims that discussing quality of life inevitably leads to devaluing the lives of groups of people associated with poor quality of life – the BMA draws a distinction between the value of the treatment and the value of the patient. It is certainly reasonable to suppose that a person can be very valuable (well loved and wanted, even) and recognise that a particular treatment will not be effective in saving their life. However, as we have already seen, effectiveness is only part of what makes a treatment beneficial. Since the value of the treatment should also be assessed in terms of resulting the quality of life of the patient, it is difficult to see how this distinction between the value of treatment and patient can be maintained. If the value of a person's life is to be found in its quality, and its quality is poor, surely the value of this life is less? One way out of this problem is to accept, as Harris does, that the value of life, whilst related to its quality, is something that can only be assessed by the person whose life it is [20]. The BMA would, however, have to resist this rescue line because of their commitment to allowing the doctor to make the final decision with regard to the benefit of treatment, even in the face of a disagreement between doctor and patient about its relative benefits and burdens.

Conclusion   Although commendable, the BMA guidelines provide less of a consensus than first appears to be the case. Whilst the principle that treatment should be withheld if it is providing no benefit is initially attractive, it is not likely to achieve a consensus in practice because the BMA assume that the value of life is attached to quality of life. This remains a contentious issue. Also, the BMA wants to separate the value of the treatment from the value of the patient, but is unable to do this as long as the value of the treatment is linked to the quality of the patient's life, and the quality of the patient's life is linked to their value of life.

Euthanasia – is consensus possible?

So far, I have shown that, as far as life-sustaining treatment in concerned, behind apparent consensus lurk several knife-edge issues. I now want to argue that, whilst no consensus is likely on the issue of euthanasia, greater consensus on withdrawing and withholding life-sustaining treatment might be possible if there was greater consensus on how the term 'euthanasia' is to be defined and applied.

Defining euthanasia

Many writers are content to define euthanasia in terms of its translation from the Greek: a good death. This is obviously an inadequate definition because it admits too many different kinds of death, most of which have nothing to do with the current debate on the rights and wrongs of euthanasia. An elderly man dying naturally in his sleep might be described as having had a good death, but there is no hint of euthanasia. Similarly, many Christians might argue that Christ, who they believed died willingly to save humankind, had the epitome of a good death, but not one that would be described as euthanasia. In order to understand what euthanasia is and is not, we need a much clear definition, one that takes account of all the morally relevant elements outlined in Chapter 1: moral agent, subject of concern, motive and intentions, means and consequences. The definition of euthanasia that will be used in this chapter is that a euthanasia occurs when one person intentionally causes the death of another person, motivated by the desire to promote the best interests of the person who dies (best interests in this context is taken to mean that they are better off dead than alive) and using the most gentle means that are available to achieve this end[24].

It is unlikely that consensus on the rights and wrongs of euthanasia will be reached because one's ethical evaluation will depend upon deep knife-edge issues, like whether killing can ever be justified and whether life has intrinsic value or whether its value is dependent upon its quality. The moral objections to withdrawing or withholding life-sustaining therapies, however, may be lightened if a consensus can be reached that some cases, that are similar to euthanasia, are not examples of euthanasia at all. Indeed, this is what the BMA has managed to achieve by concentrating attention on the fact the life-sustaining treatment is just treatment like any other. My concern is that, particularly in the context of intensive care, this principle ignores the connection between what is removed or withheld and the death of the patient. Withdrawing a ventilator may *feel*, and, therefore, seem, more like causing the death of a patient than deciding not to continue with chemotherapy. What can be described as a feeling in some cases becomes more tangibly a moral objection when it can be shown that in some cases life-sustaining treatment *is* withdrawn with the intention that the patient should die, and the debate about whether passive euthanasia is wrong (or as wrong) as active euthanasia has only served to feed the impression that all cases of withdrawing and withholding life-sustaining treatments are cases of passive euthanasia.

Two questions now need to be raised. The first is whether it is possible to ignore that fact that a patient will die as a result of treatment being withdrawn or withheld, and the second is whether the intention that the patient will die is actually behind all cases of withdrawing and withholding of life-sustaining treatments.

Acts and omissions – killing and letting die

The first question is often seen in terms of whether a distinction can be drawn between acts and omissions. If we accept, as many people do, that killing is wrong, it does not matter how the death is achieved, and this question may seem perverse as it suggests that some means of killing might be acceptable, namely those means that require us not to act. Philosophical illustrations abound. Philippa Foot, for instance, uses the example of poisoning, asking whether there is a difference between wanting someone dead and putting poison in her tea and seeing the same person spoon poison into her tea believing it to be sugar and doing nothing to stop her drinking it[25]. Rachels asks whether to hold a child one wants dead under the water until he drowns is worse than watching the same child drown in an accident and doing nothing to intervene[26]. Foot argues that the difference turns on whether any 'origination of evil' is involved (p. 287)[25]. Whilst it is undoubtedly wrong to kill someone, one can fail to rescue someone without originating the evil that causes death – though, depending upon the cost to oneself of rescuing them, one may, of course, be guilty of an appalling lack of charity or even a failure of a duty to offer protection to the vulnerable. Trammell resolves the problem in a different way. He argues that the duty to save life when we can places on our shoulders a moral duty that we cannot possible discharge completely because the demand (number of lives to be saved) is too great[27]. Rachels, along with other consequentialist writers, takes the view that we should concentrate on the outcome rather than the means, in which case allowing a child one wants dead to drown is as bad as drowning the child oneself[26].

What the views of all of these writers have in common is that they give weight to the intention behind the action or inaction. Even Rachels, the consequentialist, has to add the dimension of wanting (willing) the child to be dead. Trammell's defence of the acts/omissions distinction largely works because he assumes that we have no intention to see perish the many lives we are unable to save. Another common thread is that actions or inactions that result in human deaths are inherently more serious that those that do not. Even though Foot argues for retaining the acts and omissions distinction, she does not think that the failure to save life when one can is morally neutral. There isn't time in this chapter to attempt to resolve the acts and omissions debate (see instead Steinbock and Norcross[28]). What we have here is an illustration of the difficulties – knife-edge difficulties – that the BMA has tended to sweep under the carpet by giving life-sustaining treatment the same status as any other kind of treatment.

Some causing of death is not euthanasia – the role of intention, motive, means and cause

One argument for retaining the acts and omission doctrine is that, without it, many omissions would be given the same moral status as actions or, in the medical context, withdrawing life-sustaining treatment would be the same as killing the patient. This is a view that has its own supporters, like those who sponsored the Private Members' Bill intended to compel doctors not to withdraw or withhold life-sustaining treatment. It is, however, possible to argue for something midway between the position of the BMA (that life-sustaining treatment should be viewed as no different from any other kind of treatment) and the Private Members' Bill (that would have us act as though any decision to withdraw or withhold life-sustaining treatment should be treated as tantamount to murder). This argument focuses more closely on the intentions and motives of acts and omissions.

Intentions and motives   Rachels' argument that there is no distinction between active and passive euthanasia is compelling, partly because it is a highly qualified example of the acts/omissions debate. The qualification is that it applies to euthanasia. We already distinguish between different kinds of causing death, and these distinctions sometimes operate to condone some forms of causing death or to indicate that different levels of punishment should be applied. So, for instance, we distinguish between causing the death of another person and causing one's own death; we distinguish murder from euthanasia (even if the law does not); we recognise that murder and capital punishment are different even if we disapprove of capital punishment; we recognise a difference between manslaughter and murder; and so forth. According to my definition, euthanasia is the intentional causing of death motivated by best interests. Even supporters of euthanasia agree that it requires the intentional causing of death, but what distinguishes euthanasia from murder is that it is motivated by benevolence.

The law makes no such distinction between intention and motive but moral philosophy does. For instance, imagine a situation in which a rich elderly man is terminally ill, dying slowly and in intractable pain. Imagine further that his nurse gives him, at his request, a massive dose of morphine to cause his death. This sounds very like euthanasia until we add to the account the fact that the nurse was not motivated by the man's plight but by the fact that she stood to inherit a fortune from his estate. Irrespective of the fact that the elderly man had the blessed release from life that he requested, this was not euthanasia because it was not benevolently motivated. Imagine a similar situation, only this time the nurse does not stand to inherit and she also does not approve of euthanasia. However, when administering the pain relief, she miscalculates the dose and, in error, gives the patient a fatal dose. In this case we may think that the death was still a good thing, or we may think that the nurse was negligent and guilty of manslaughter, but we would be unlikely to described her error as a euthanasia because there was no intention to cause the patient's death. So, when Rachels[26] sets up a scenario where there is an intention to cause the death of a baby with severe Down's syndrome and an intestinal blockage that will not, therefore, be operated upon, and he tells us that the motive is the baby's best interests, whether or not we agree with euthanasia we have to accept that it really doesn't matter how the baby's death is caused, be this by act or omission. If we disagree with euthanasia, we will condemn the death whatever the means, and if we agree with euthanasia we will think that both ways of causing the baby's death are acceptable (though we may be inclined to agree with Rachels that, once committed to euthanasia, we should chose the most gentle means available, which, in the case as he outlines it, means active euthanasia using a fatal injection).

So we ought, as Rachels suggests, draw no distinction between active and passive euthanasia even if we are not sure whether we would be prepared to reject the general distinction between acts and omissions. It then becomes important to know whether any particular withdrawing or withholding of treatment is euthanasia or not. It is important for people who disagree with euthanasia to do so, because they should condemn such omissions, and it is important for people who want euthanasia to be legalised because these kinds of omissions should be included in all of the relevant legislative changes that they propose. It also matters to practitioners because euthanasia is currently illegal, and they should know whether a decision to withdraw treatment is, therefore, also illegal.

A withdrawal or withholding of life-sustaining treatment is a euthanasia if it is withdrawn or withheld with the intention that the patient will die, and if this intention is motivated by the view that it is in the patient's best interests to be dead. Accordingly, there is a very fine line between passive euthanasia and withdrawing treatment that is thought not to benefit a patient because their quality of life is very poor. Similarly, where an effective treatment is withheld because the burden of continuing to live seems to outweigh the benefit of more life. This line is a fine one because it requires us to suppose that the doctor's sole intention is to assess the appropriateness of the treatment and that there is no intention to release the patient from a life that has such a poor quality that treatment to enable it to continue is not considered beneficial.

Cause and means Decisions to withdraw or withhold futile procedures cannot be associated with euthanasia provided that a tight definition of futility is applied. Where futility means 'will fail to achieve its physiological objective', the element of *causing* death is absent – if the procedure is futile, death would occur whether or not it is performed, and because it is futile, it can hardly be described as treatment or therapy.

There is some disagreement, however, over what counts as futility. Some definitions of futility include possibilities beyond the failure of the physiological objective: for instance, that there is only a small chance of achieving the medical objective, or that the patient cannot benefit from the physiological benefit because his or her quality of life is so poor. These types of definition come closer to crossing the line between withdrawal of treatment and euthanasia because both come close to saying that death might be preferable to continued life.

Finally, whilst the circumstances that require them to do so are regrettable, doctors must be able to withdraw or withhold treatment from one patient because it will achieve greater benefit for another. It is sometimes argued that in an intensive care unit (ICU) this is unacceptable because the patient from whom the treatment is withdrawn will die. On the other hand, it is precisely because the stakes for everyone are so high that the doctors must be free to rescue the patient with the best chance of survival. Clearly, this is not euthanasia because there is no intention that that either patient will die (despite the fact that the death of one of them is foreseeable), and nor is it motivated by the best interests of the patient who actually dies – on the contrary, the decision to remove therapy is motivated by the desire to save a different patient. The problem here is that the usual symmetry between withholding and withdrawing life-sustaining treatment is less convincing when it is applied to examples of scarcity. In non-medical cases of limited resources, it seems more acceptable to chose who is rescued than it is to sacrifice one person in order to save another. For example, withholding treatment could be compared to rowing a rescue boat to the nearest drowning person or to the person who is, otherwise, most likely to survive. But then, in a similar comparison, withdrawing treatment seems like throwing a very ill person out of the lifeboat to make room for another person who, whilst ill, seems more likely to survive. This is obviously less of a problem for consequentialists because, in both cases, the best outcome is achieved. But for others, the distinction between foreseeing and intending becomes too close for comfort. The alternatives are, however, equally unpalatable. One can continue to treat the person who is most likely to die (decline to throw them overboard) or one can put overboard someone who is marginally less ill and let them swim alongside the boat, possibly swapping now and then with other less ill people on board. This latter kind of behaviour is common in an ICU where, in order to make an urgent admission, a patient who is doing relatively well is transferred off the unit even though they are not really ready to go, in the hope that they will manage with rather less help. Of course, the discharged patient may have to be readmitted in the near future, or may even die as a result, but their death is less imminent than that of the patient who will die if they are not admitted, or the one who will certainly die if they are removed from a ventilator. A calculated risk is thereby taken with the life of the less ill patient. This policy seems rather perverse, though, because it risks the lives of those most able to survive – patients who, by analogy, were also in the lifeboat at the time when the more seriously ill patient needed to be rescued. If the important principle is that no one should lose their place in the lifeboat, then this practice is just as questionable as the one that removes the most seriously ill patient.

Conclusion

I have argued that whilst there is significant consensus on withdrawing and withholding life-sustaining treatment, this consensus can serve to obscure significant points of disagreement. Achieving consensus in some of these areas seems unlikely because it would require the wholesale reconciliation between opposing philosophical views on causing death and saving life, acts and omission, the possibility of justified killing and so forth. The consensus on withdrawing and withholding treatment is, however, useful when it comes to distinguishing some kinds of causing death from euthanasia. But, it should not be surprising if, whilst providing a legal umbrella for doctors viz. *Bolam*, the BMA guidelines do not resolve tensions between team members in ICUs. The problem of conflicts between teams is discussed elsewhere (Chapter 12), but my conclusion is that, whilst it is important for all staff to be aware of consensus documents and court rulings, they also need to remain well versed in the underlying obstacles to complete consensus, if only to understand the difficulties that some of their colleagues may still have in applying such guidance.

References

1. Kipnis K. Professional ethics and instructional success. In: Professing Medicine. A. Kao, ed. American Medical Association, 2001
2. *Bolam v. Friern Hospital Management Committee* [1957] 1 WLR 582

3.   General Medical Council. Withholding and Withdrawing Life-prolonging Treatments: Good Practice in Decision making. London: GMC, 2002
4.   British Medical Association. Withholding and Withdrawing Life-Prolonging Medical Treatment. 2nd edn. London: BMA Publishing, 2001
5.   *Airedale NHS Trust v. Bland* [1993] 1 All ER 821
6.   *Re B (Adult: refusal of medical treatment)* [2002] 2 All England Law Reports 449
7.   Draper H. Anorexia Nervosa and respecting a refusal of life-prolonging therapy: a limited justification. Bioethics 2000; 14: 120–33
8.   *Re MB* [1997] 2 FLR 426
9.   *St George's Healthcare NHS Trust v. S* [1998] 3 WLR 936
10. *Sidaway v. Bethlem RHG* [1985] 1 All ER 666
11. Montgomery J. Health Care Law. Oxford: Oxford University Press, 1997
12. Kennedy, I. Treat Me Right. Oxford: Clarendon Press, 1988
13. Biggs H. I don't want to be a burden! A feminist reflects on women's experiences of death and dying. In: Feminist Perspectives on Health Care Law. S. Sheldon, M. Thomson, eds. London: Cavendish Publishing, 1998: 279–95
14. Draper H, Sorell T. Patients' responsibilities medical ethics. Bioethics 2002; 16: 335–52
15. Buchanan A, Brock D. Deciding for Others. Cambridge: Cambridge University Press, 1989
16. Wicclair MR. Patient decision-making, capacity and risk. Bioethics 1991; 5: 91–104
17. *Frenchy NHS Trust v. S* [1994] 2 All ER 403
18. *Practice Note (Vegetative State)* [1996] 2 FLR 375
19. Royal College of Physicians. Guidelines on the diagnosis and management of the permanent vegetative state. J Royal Coll Physicians 1996; 30: 119–21
20. Harris J. The Value of Life. Routledge Kegan Paul, 1985
21. Glover J. Causing Death and Saving Lives. Penguin, 1977
22. Singer P. Rethinking Life and Death. Oxford: Oxford University Press, 1998
23. Nagel T. Death: Mortal Questions. Cambridge: Cambridge University Press, 1979
24. Draper H. Euthanasia. In: Encyclopaedia of Applied Ethics. R. Chadwick, ed. London: Academic Press, 1998
25. Foot P. Killing and letting die. In: Killing and Letting Die. B. Steinbock, A. Norcross, eds. Fordham University Press, 1994: 287
26. Rachels J. Active and Passive Euthanasia. In: Applied Ethics. P. Singer, ed. Oxford: Oxford University Press, 1986: 29–35
27. Trammell R. Saving life and taking life. In: Killing and Letting Die. B. Steinbock, A. Norcross, eds. Fordham University Press, 1994: 290–7
28. Steinbock B, Norcross A. eds. Killing and Letting Die. Fordham University Press, 1994

Brain Death and the Cadaveric Organ Donor

14

David Lamb

Introduction

The post-mortem management of brain-dead organ donors continues to generate controversy and scepticism regarding the reliability of criteria and tests for brain death. It will be argued here that, while there have not been any developments in medical science to invalidate the concept and criteria for brain death[1–3], one of the primary reasons for public unease is the manner in which medical technology has contributed to a transformation in the management of the cadaveric organ donor.

Objections to brain-related criteria for death

Since the early 1970s, medical authorities, supported by governments in Europe and the USA, have endorsed neurological criteria for the determination of death. Nevertheless, scepticism with regard to the reliability of the tests for brain death, and criticism of the linkage with organ transplantation has persisted. This has occasionally burst into a major scandal, such as the one, in the UK, following the BBC's broadcast in 1980, which alleged that the brain-dead were not really dead[4]. Throughout the 1990s, Germany encountered a fierce debate over the status of brain death and criteria for organ retrieval. In 1996, the German Parliament considered revising their statute to make criteria for diagnosing brain death more stringent. In 1997, after a lengthy debate, the German Parliament passed laws that adopted existing practice throughout Europe. At the root of the problem were public perceptions regarding the management of donor bodies.

During the summer of 2000, the debate on brain death erupted in the United Kingdom when several anaesthetists called for the administration of anaesthetics to brain-dead organ donors prior to organ removal, giving rise to speculation that 'dead' donors could be experiencing pain, and that there was residual life in patients after a diagnosis of brainstem death. It was reported that some doctors anaesthetised organ donors after the diagnosis of death before removing their organs. The claim that EEG readings were detectable in brainstem dead preparations also resurfaced, despite more than 30 years of evidence that post-mortem electrical activity is not a valid indicator of life. Replying to the debate, Giles Morgan, President of the UK's Intensive Care Society, said that, while electrical activity can be perceived in some parts of the brain when the brainstem is dead, 'it is disorganised random electricity. The whole brain is functionally disintegrating' (p. 1)[5].

A report in the *Guardian* newspaper said that many anaesthetists 'confess to lingering doubts as to what might be still happening in the brain of the donor, even though his or her brainstem shows no response to tests and there is no question of survival – even on a life-support machine – for more than a few days' (p. 1)[5]. One might note the confusing terminology where 'life-support' enhances 'survival' for a 'few days' after brainstem death. No alternative concept of death was cited, and no reference was made to scientific evidence to justify 'lingering doubts' regarding the possibility of brain activity in a brain that has been thoroughly tested for any signs of life. One might infer that whatever is functioning with the assistance of technology meets the author's concept of life. Consequently any movement in the body, such as spinal chord reflexes, post-mortem muscular contractions, or change in pulse or blood pressure during the artificial maintenance of the body, would also be cited as evidence of persistent life. As brain-dead preparations are maintained for the purpose of organ transplantation, opponents of brain-related concepts for death might argue that criteria for brainstem death is merely a means of obtaining organs before the patient is really dead. What being 'really dead' actually means is not explicitly stated.

The unease experienced by some anaesthetists cited in the British media is, nevertheless, understandable from a common-sense point of view, especially if philosophical issues regarding the definition of death have not been addressed. With a living patient, it is normal to provide an anaesthetic before administering a paralysing drug that prevents muscular contractions. Under certain circumstances, transplant surgeons will request that a paralysing drug will be given to brain-dead individuals to prevent muscular contraction. Since the brain-dead in these circumstances appear to mimic the living, and respond to surgical intervention in ways that mimic the living, several anaesthetists have accordingly administered an anaesthetic prior to organ removal. These interventions, which are said to be distressing to nurses and medical personnel, are by-products of the technology employed to maintain transplantable organs. Consequently, expressions of unease are said to have an adverse effect on the transplant programme. In such an atmosphere, where anaesthetists claim that they have been 'reluctant to speak publicly for fear of damaging the transplant programme' (p. 1)[5], there is little scope for consideration of the philosophical proposal that brainstem death is death in its own right.

As part of a programme for managing donor cadavers, the administration of anaesthetics prior to organ removal cannot benefit the donor, but when it is portrayed as a benefit to the donor, the proposal to anaesthetise brain-dead individuals prior to organ removal has serious ethical implications. Superficially, it sounds like an extra precaution that would not harm the donor. One consultant anaesthetist called for anaesthetics to be 'routinely given to all donors diagnosed as brain dead', adding 'that such a step would bring forward more donors' (p. 4)[6], thereby baiting the proposal with utilitarian benefit. This implies that the brainstem dead are not really dead. If they can feel pain, they are not dead. But, if they are not dead, they could not be cadaveric donors, and any proposal to give them anaesthetics to relieve pain is an admission that organs are being removed from the living, which is obviously immoral, and accordingly anaesthetists should not be involved with such practices.

Brain death and the donor controversy

One of the most persistent lines of criticism of brain-related criteria for death is bound up with its alleged interconnectedness with organ transplantation. According to one critic, Peter McCullagh, 'it is likely that the determination of death and organ transplantation will remain intertwined in the future' (p. 1)[7]. McCullagh, however, recognises that: '(w)hilst the definition of the state of brain death occurred independently of the process of identifying prospective organ donors, attitudes towards both brain dead and the management of individuals diagnosed as brain dead have been influenced by the concurrent development of transplant surgery' (p. 8)[7]. McCullagh is clearly correct to insist that brain death originated as a need to limit treatment to patients who were beyond any benefit from treatment, but he is on weaker ground when he argues that the management of donors has influenced criteria for brain death. Quite obviously, techniques for the post-mortem management of donors have developed with the interests of organ retrieval in mind (and this may give rise to ethical concern regarding what it is considered appropriate to do to dead bodies), but this need not erode the principle that the management of the dying donor should be unrelated to the interests of the potential recipient.

The aggressive maintenance of the brain-dead, which may include the employment of cardiopulmonary resuscitation, is nevertheless suggestive that procedures to maintain the living are in continuance until a decision is taken to withdraw ventilatory support. In fact, several commentators have stressed similarities between therapy provided for the dying and techniques for managing brain-dead donors for the purpose of maintaining transplantable organs in optimal conditions. The inference that is frequently drawn is that criteria for brain death is an arbitrary matter designed to facilitate the processes associated with organ retrieval. It must be stressed that, as the medical technology improves, management of the brain-dead will produce even stronger signs of life. None of these techniques should be interpreted as means of preserving life in the brain-dead. From the moment brainstem death has occurred, it must be recognised that the body is 'trying to die' and that dead donor management is the attempt to prevent or delay the many physiological changes that take place when the brain ceases to function. Consequently, techniques used to retain life are also employed for the maintenance of organs. For example, cardiopulmonary resuscitation is employed to restart a heart in a cadaver. Numerous chemical technologies can substitute for normal functions. 'Breathing, blood pressure, temperature control, fluid and electrolyte balance and hormone production must be managed externally. The lungs, brachia and stomach must be suctioned routinely to remove excess fluids' (p. 150)[8]. Even units of blood may be replaced. Antibiotics may be given to ward off infection, and a variety of pharmaceutical agents may be circulated through the body to replace fluid and maintain the balance in physiological systems. In this context, Linda F. Hogle (p. 152)[8] refers to the maintenance of 'donor cyborgs', where the body becomes a new type of 'human–technology composite'. She refers to new pharmaceutical agents that can go beyond donor maintenance, and will be designed to preserve cell integrity, inhibit certain functions and encourage others. Organs can actually be improved – made more resilient – while being worked upon in the donor's body. In this context Hogle (p. 152)[8] speaks of 'donor enhancement'. All of this gives the impression that a living person is being cared for. The objective, however, is not the prolonged treatment of patients but the production of 'prime quality organs'. Some may argue that it manifests a lack of respect for the dead, others may see it as a rational use of society's resources.

In a critical review of brain-related criteria for death and organ retrieval, Nora Machado draws attention to public uncertainties regarding the status of the brain-dead organ donor, pointing out that some medical personnel and many next of kin do not see the brain-dead as unequivocally in the category of the dead[9]. This cannot be denied, and it must be acknowledged that medical technology is out of step with public perceptions of death[10]. Perhaps there is scope for philosophical reflection on a distinction between 'being dead' and 'being lifeless'. For some, so it appears, the brain-dead are dead, but not lifeless. People still associate death with a lifeless cold body, not with a warm, perspiring, brain-dead preparation. Even the fact that the brain-dead are maintained in intensive care units is suggestive of continuing life that is being 'cared' for. But confusion between the living and the dead, in such cases, must be met with clarity. Unfortunately Machado's discussion of the moral dilemmas of brain death only adds to current feelings of uncertainty. While most medical personnel, she argues, would have no objections to extracting organs from the brain-dead, 'only for the purpose of helping another person . . . the thought of . . . cremating a brain dead with sustained circulation and breathing would be regarded by most as morally revolting' (p. 98)[9].

The problem with this line of argument is that it perpetuates the (mistaken) belief that neurological criteria for death is primarily for the benefit of organ recipients; whereas its primary purpose is to indicate the point at which it is morally appropriate to cease treating a patient and initiate what is morally appropriate behaviour towards a corpse. Her reference to the cremation of a being with circulation and breathing merely compounds confusion with misleading imagery: a brain-dead ex-patient could only be cremated in such a fashion if the ventilator was included in the process, which would be a morally revolting waste of resources! Machado cites numerous sources that record feelings of uncertainty regarding brain death, usually in the context of relatives noting the appearance of life. These are clearly examples where a professional response to cultural meanings attached to life and death requires sensitivity. But nowhere does Machado cite well-documented reversals of brain death. Trails of confusion are also laid with reference to the brain-dead being kept alive on ventilators, and citing nurses who say that the patient 'suffered brain death and died the next day', also referring to 'extended life' after 'cerebral death', hinting of diagnostic inaccuracy regarding the reliability of EEG measurements and tests for blood circulation in the brain, neither of which are essential nor mandatory for a diagnosis of death.

Scepticism regarding the diagnosis of death is frequently expressed in misleading descriptions of post-mortem donor management. In discussions that pay no regard to the appropriate concept and criteria for death expressions like 'he is brain-dead, but we have just performed successful cardiopulmonary resuscitation' or 'The brain-dead patient has been put on a course of antibiotics', are suggestive that a patient (as opposed to the parts of a corpse) is being cared for. Expressions to the effect that one is brain dead and being maintained on a 'life support machine', which one 'chooses' to 'turn off' is probably the most common source of confusion. Further confusion is manifest when the brain-dead are referred to as 'living cadavers' because of the extension of artificial feeding and mechanical support. One frequently cited remark was made by a judge in Florida when he said: 'This Lady is dead and has been dead and she is being kept alive artificially.'[11]

Should the definition and criteria for death be a matter of personal choice?

Since the early 1970s, most countries have opted for statutes or legally endorsed guidelines for the determination of death but, during periods of controversy regarding the criteria for death, proposals have emerged whereby the determination of death should be a matter for the individual. During the 1990s, such was the hostility to the existing criteria for brain death that the German Green Party put forward a recommendation that every individual should provide their own definition of death and, somehow, record this information in a central registry. The American bioethicist, Robert M. Veatch, who has for many years maintained that death should be equated with the persistent vegetative state (which he describes as a 'higher brain definition'), has also argued in favour of a personal definition of death[12]. Veatch's argument is based on his belief that the debate over a definition of death is primarily a moral one and that, as we are not likely to reach consensus on such moral questions, the imposition of one moral view over others tramples on an individual's capacity for moral dissent. So, argues Veatch, diversity must be tolerated as long as it does not cause insurmountable problems for others, such as a threat to public health. Within this tolerable range would be higher brain definitions based on irreversible loss of the capacity for consciousness.

Apart from the problems that personal definitions would create regarding hospital routines, such as a massive infrastructure required to give every individual equal preferences, there would be several interesting ramifications. One

pregnant and her doctors decided to maintain her body in an attempt to preserve the life of the foetus. Earlier attempts at post-mortem maternal ventilation had involved more fully developed foetuses that could very soon be viable on their own. By 1992, the limits of artificial support that could be provided for the organs within a brain-dead body far exceeded earlier forecasts, but the continued management of a brain-dead body had not been attempted for as long as the Erlangen proposal envisaged. From the outset, critics saw it as an experiment to test the very limits of medical technology. In the event the 'Erlangen Experiment', as it was called by the media, created a major controversy, raising both criticism and questions regarding the status of brain-related criteria for death. Public reaction was hostile, and this hostility generated thousands of publications expressing scepticism regarding brain death.

The source of the controversy could be seen in the chemical and mechanical technologies employed to maintain the woman's body in its brain dead state (pp. 80–1)[8]. It is instructive to consider these technologies from the point of view of a lay person trying to understand modern medicine's criteria for drawing the boundary between life and death. Although the doctors insisted that it was a corpse that was being maintained, the battery of therapeutic interventions were suggestive of attempts to maintain a living being. Artificial nutrition was provided, giving rise to philosophical and ethical questions regarding the possibility and desirability of feeding a corpse. Hormones were administered, thus maintaining a 'normal' state of pregnancy. When the kidneys began to fail, dialysis was initiated. One of the woman's eyes became infected and it was removed. Antibiotics were not infused out of concern for the foetus. A foetus requires maternal exercise, so the body was moved as if it were exercising, and other activities were provided to give a natural setting. Music was played and nurses reported that the foetus 'is happy when it hears beautiful music' (p. 80)[8].

These measures were not directed at the prolongation of maternal life; the objective was to provide a safe environment for the foetus. But, for the lay person, it was hard to comprehend a distinction between the management of a very sick mother and a brain-dead preparation that was being used as an incubator.

This problem repeatedly surfaced during the 1980s and 1990s, where public perceptions of death as a wholly lifeless state conflicted with brain-related criteria for death and the management of corpses in intensive care units. With hindsight, it is important to concede that lay objections to brain death are not rebutted with accusations of ignorance regarding medical facts – which is an appropriate method for dealing with a sceptical clinician – but by understanding prevailing cultural beliefs about death[10]. The public outcry over the 'Erlangen Experiment' revealed the extent to which scientific medicine is at variance with cultural opinions about death. Questions concerning the status of brain death have often been resolved with reassurances that 'brain death' means that the loss of certain brain functions *is* death of the whole person, including both brain and body, and that post-mortem management of the brain-dead is merely a brief moment before the removal of organs that would inevitably perish within a short time. But now, it appeared obvious to all that the dead body contained life that could be maintained indefinitely. In the event, the foetus aborted after six weeks, and even the way this fact was presented generated confusion, with references to the mother being 'turned off' after the death of the foetus.

From a philosophical perspective, the problem was created through not attending to the important distinction between death of the whole body (which would be putrefaction and meaningless as a concept of death) and death of the body as a whole, which stresses integration and organisation. It was never acknowledged that what occurs in brain death is death of the body as a whole, not death or even imminent death, of every component. Confusion was compounded with references to 'ongoing life' in the body, yet the very fact that viable organs and tissues can be taken from either the brain-dead or victims of irreversible cardiac arrest is clear evidence that death is not equated with death of the whole body.

There were several legal and political issues in the Erlangen case that had not been raised in the earlier discussions of maternal ventilation in the USA a decade earlier. Although Marian Ploch's physicians had diagnosed her as brain dead the coroner refused to sign a death certificate, insisting that the baby would be born without a mother, which was held to be a technical impossibility. As Hogle said: 'She was legally but not officially dead' (p. 81)[8]. Various interest groups saw the Erlangen experiment as a battlefield. Pro- and anti-abortion campaigners took their respective stands over the application of the technology, and the status of brain death became a battlefield between the authority of medical scientists and the rights of ordinary citizens. Doubts regarding the status of brain death were given widespread publicity, which resurfaced in the debate on brain death in the German Parliament in 1996, and the case continues to generate controversy with regard to brain death and cadaveric organ donation.

The separation principle

It is important, both scientifically and morally, to maintain a clear separation between the concept and criteria for death on the one hand and extraneous factors on the other hand. Matters relating to the cost of therapy, poor prognosis, quality of life, arguments for euthanasia, and the need to procure transplant organs are all fundamentally distinct from criteria for death. Criteria for death must be exclusively linked to the condition of the patient. Therefore, proposals to classify patients in persistent vegetative states, or anencephalic infants with functioning brainstems, as dead, for the purpose of early organ removal, seriously confuse arguments about the definition of death with extraneous needs. Similar objections apply to proposals for additional confirmatory tests, or the administration of anaesthetics to brain-dead patients prior to organ removal in order to promote confidence in the transplant programme. The case for brainstem death as death in its own right should not involve attempts to deceive the public with irrelevant confirmatory tests or persuasion based on the utilitarian benefits of organ transplantation. Too often, proponents of brain-oriented definitions of death have spoken of the benefits of harvesting organs from brain-dead donors. Consequently, their opponents have gone on to accuse them of gerrymandering the definition of death in order to facilitate early organ removal.

201

It should be stressed that consideration of organ donation should come second to basic medical management. This should be unaffected by a patient's autonomous desire to donate organs. A common criticism of brainstem death is that an interest in organ procurement puts pressure on neurologists and neuro-surgeons to redefine death. This is not the case. In the 1950s, long before cardiac transplantation, when renal transplants were highly experimental and conducted only on genetically identical twins with massive irradiation of the recipient, there were profound ethical discussions concerning the value of ventilation to asystole when treatment for patients in irreversible apnoeic coma was obviously hopeless and increasingly gruesome.

To maintain independence of brain-related criteria for death it is, therefore, important that statutes and guidelines for brain death should specify that the primary interest in formulating a definition of death is to recognise a morally significant boundary between the duties owed to a living patient and those that are appropriate to a corpse. Any baiting of the definition of death with extraneous benefits will only taint the scientific purity of the case for brain death and introduce the notion that an individual's death can be determined by societal needs. Suggestions that more stringent tests be conducted when organ transplantation is envisaged involve a public relations exercise which should be resisted, as it forges an unnecessary link between criteria for death and the requirement for organs. It is misleading to propose either looser or more stringent criteria for diagnosing the death of organ donors, as this would entail the absurd suggestion that there is a special kind of death awaiting them.

When tests have clearly indicated brain death, it must be recognised that treatment of the patient has ceased, no matter what actions are performed upon the corpse. Conventionally, the determination of death was followed by the act of drawing a sheet over the corpse and initiating actions associated with proper disposal of the remains. A clear-cut line separates the two activities. There is a moral imperative to classify or define a person as dead or alive, as the consequences of such a decision affect actions towards that individual. It is immoral to treat the living as dead, and it is also immoral to treat the dead as alive. When death marks the boundary between the cessation of therapy for the dying and the initiation of procedures associated with transplantation, there is a moral requirement for a *principle of separation*. Thus, practices and, indeed, laws have emerged that require a different institutional framework for dealing with the treatment of the dying and the management of a corpse. In most European countries, there are laws and regulations that stipulate that the physician in charge of a patient waiting for a transplant organ cannot determine the death status of a potential donor or be involved in the extraction of particular organs. This avoids a conflict of interests on the part of doctors and safeguards the rights of seriously ill or dying patients.

In practice, however, referral to the transplant team from the intensive care unit may involve a necessary amount of collaboration. In such circumstances, there is a shift in attitudes towards the potential donor following a diagnosis of brain death. Linda F. Hogle recalls an experience in the USA where she noted that:

. . . the potential donor had a distinct identity as a person up to the time the doctors determined that he was probably brain dead and thus a potential organ donor. From this point, there was a continual shift through the process of determining eligibility and the right to use bodily materials up to the time of procurement itself. As soon as brain death was declared, procurement personnel dropped any reference to the person as a patient and ceased using the patient's name. He was thereafter referred to by cause of death, age, or hospital location or simply as the donor; for example, a brain dead patient may be called 'the twenty-four-year-old-drive-by shooting at the General Hospital. (p. 142)[8]

This change in attitudes reflects, perhaps, the most important ethical principle in transplantation ethics – the principle of separation – which requires a distinction between duties appropriate to the dying and procedures associated with the disposal of the corpse, *and that management of the dying donor should not be influenced by the interests of the potential recipient.*

Conclusion

Sophisticated technology in intensive care units has confronted us with a need to understand and define death. Sophisticated means of maintaining potential transplant organs in the bodies of the deceased has, however, created public anxiety. It is important that this anxiety is not manipulated into a form of scepticism regarding criteria for death. Perhaps it is time to consider whether the intrusion of science into the management of brain-dead bodies has gone beyond what is regarded as morally acceptable behaviour towards a corpse. The view that requirements for transplantable organs determines criteria for brain death must be combated. If transplant surgery were outlawed, if a supply of artificial organs eliminated all need for human cadaver organs, if the costs of maintaining patients for indefinitely prolonged periods in intensive care units were dramatically reduced, there would still be a need for precise guidelines on brain death. The need for a definition of death is a by-product of medical science, and objective criteria for death are essential for the cessation of therapy, but the primary reason in formulating objective criteria must be strictly limited to the interests of the dying individual.

References

1. Lamb D. Transplante de Orgãos Ética. São Paulo: Editora Hucitec, 2000
2. Lamb D. Etica, Morte E Morte Encefalica. São Paulo: Office Editora e Publicidade Ltda, 2001
3. Pallis C. Brainstem death. In: Vinken PJ, Bruyn GW, Klawans HL, eds. Coedited by Braakman R. Handbook of Clinical Neurology Vol. 57, Revised series 13, Head Injury. Amsterdam: Elsevier, 1990: 441–96
4. BBC, Panorama. 13 October 1980
5. Boseley S. Doctors call for anaesthetics for brainstem-dead donors. The Guardian, 19 August 2000
6. Keep P. quoted by R. Allison. Brain death debate may deter organ donors. The Guardian, 21 August 2000:4
7. McCullagh In: Brain Dead, Brain Absent, Brain Donors. Chichester: John Wiley, 1993

203

8. Hogle LF. Recovering the Nations' Body. New Brunswick: Rutgers University Press, 1999
9. Machado N. Using the Bodies of the Dead. Aldershot: Ashgate, 1999
10. Gill P. Brainstem death – an anthropological perspective. Care Crit Ill 2000; 16: 217–20
11. Anon. Life-support ended, a woman dies. New York Times, 5 December 1976
12. Veatch RM. Transplantation Ethics. Washington: Georgetown University Press, 2000
13. Smith DR. Legal recognition of neocortical death. Cornell Law Review, 1986; 71: 850–88
14. Parisi JE, Kim RC, Collins GH, Hillinger MF. Brain death with prolonged somatic survival. N Engl J Med 1982; 306: 14–16
15. Pallis C. Return to Elsinore. J Med Ethics 1990; 16: 10–12
16. Field DR, Gates EA, Creasy RK, Jonsen AR Lares RK. Maternal brain death during pregnancy. JAMA, 1988; 248: 1089–91
17. Siegler M, Wikler D. Brain Death and Live Birth [Editorial]. JAMA, 1982; 248: 1101–2

The Acceptability of Routine Testing for Blood-borne Communicable Diseases 15

Rebecca Bennett

Introduction

Since the early 1970s, there has been a move away from the traditional approach to the control of communicable disease. The emphasis now is usually on patient autonomy rather than coercive containment and treatment. There are clear reasons for this. These reasons include the central role patient autonomy has come to occupy in health care and the impact that HIV/AIDS has had in revolutionising policy in the area of communicable disease control. Whereas covert and even coercive testing and treatment was often an accepted part of traditional disease control, it is now generally accepted that competent individuals should be allowed to choose whether or not to have diagnostic tests, especially those that may indicate potentially serious conditions. While there may be temptations on the part of health professionals to test for conditions without the explicit informed consent of patients[1] such temptations are usually deemed unacceptably paternalistic. However, with the continued increase of HIV and hepatitis infections and the re-emergence of forgotten infections, such as tuberculosis and diphtheria, the increase of air travel, the increased number of immuno-suppressed patients and epidemics involving antibiotic-resistant stains of infectious disease, there are those who argue that patient autonomy is standing in the way of disease control[2].

This chapter looks at current policy as it relates to communicable disease control and asks whether policy based on the principle of respect for patient autonomy is appropriate in light of the threats that face us in terms of existing, new and resistant forms of communicable disease. In particular, this chapter considers whether widespread testing of patients undergoing invasive treatment, or of health-care professionals involved in exposure-prone procedures, may be ethically justifiable. If this widespread testing aimed to achieve a high uptake of these tests within these groups, these tests could no longer be considered fully voluntary.

Any testing regimen where there is a level of coercion would, of course, infringe an individual's autonomy but, arguably, for good reasons – in order to minimise further infection. There is precedent for infringing individual autonomy in order to protect third parties from infection, not only in draconian legislation established within an earlier tradition of public health policy (e.g. *UK Public Health (Control of Diseases) Act 1984*) but also in contemporary measures such as routine antenatal HIV testing. This chapter asks if it justifiable to routinely test specific groups in society, such as pregnant women, for serious communicable diseases and whether this precedent lends support for routine testing of other groups, such as patients undergoing invasive procedures or health-care professionals involved in exposure-prone practices. What is the role of individual autonomy in a clinical environment where transmission of serious communicable diseases is a real, if remote, risk, and is there a case for saying that some people's autonomy is more sacred than others?

Autonomy, HIV and policy

Patient autonomy is increasingly, and rightly, perceived as a manifestation of the individual's rights of self-determination and privacy, universally regarded as a pillar of civil liberty, and this is reflected in legal and social policy as well as ethical doctrine.* While there may be temptations on the part of medical professionals to intervene to protect individuals from their health-care choices, it is usually accepted that if these choices can be deemed autonomous then they must be respected, regardless of the possible adverse consequences of such action; to do otherwise would be unjustified paternalism. If one holds that respect for individual autonomy is important, one does so because this freedom to orchestrate one's own life is an important factor in making a life valuable. An individual cannot have this valuable freedom if only the choices others believe to be beneficial are allowed.

In line with the development of this central role of the rights of the patient, when policy was developed to cope with the emergence of HIV in the mid-1980s there was a tendency to treat HIV/AIDS differently than other communicable diseases. Instead of the traditional approach to communicable disease control, policy relating to HIV and AIDS tends to emphasise medical confidentiality, individual autonomy and informed consent. This tendency to treat those with HIV/AIDS differently than individuals with other communicable diseases has been described as 'HIV/AIDS exceptionalism'[3]. Before therapeutic interventions became available, it appeared that there was little to be gained by coercive HIV policies. People were unable to change the course of their disease if they were infected, and it was unclear that knowledge of one's HIV-positive status had any effect on behaviour. Unlike other communicable diseases, HIV could only be transmitted by intimate contact with an infected individual. It was, therefore,

---

* See for example the European Convention on Human Rights details of which can be found under Convention for the Protection of Human Rights and Fundamental Freedoms at http://conventions.coe.int/treaty/EN/cadreprincipal.htm.

possible for the uninfected to protect themselves and for the infected to protect others without necessarily being tested for HIV. Therefore, coercive testing regimes would not only be ethically problematic in terms of individual rights but also possibly ineffective in the prevention of further infection. It was felt that the best approach involved the protection of the rights of those infected in order that people would feel confident to come forward for testing and advice. It was thought that behaviour change would be best facilitated in a non-coercive atmosphere.

While this approach sits more easily with the current emphasis on respect for individual autonomy, it has led to worries concerning the effect this approach may have in terms of controlling the spread of HIV and controlling other communicable diseases. While there are those who welcome this emphasis on patient autonomy, which was in part established by the response to HIV, there are others who argue that the 'exceptionalist' approach to HIV not only should *not* be expanded to other serious communicable diseases but should be *repealed* in the case of HIV/AIDS.

It has been argued that while treating HIV in this unconventional way may have been the most appropriate approach before recent therapeutic interventions were available, now these interventions are available, earlier and widespread diagnosis of HIV infection becomes a priority. If HIV is diagnosed in its early stages it may be possible, using therapeutic interventions, to influence the clinical course of infection and, in pregnant women, possibly reduce the risk of perinatal transmission. However, in order to increase early diagnosis of HIV, it is argued that HIV should be treated more like other infectious diseases, allowing the implementation of more widespread testing and screening programmes. In this way it is hoped that more people will be 'encouraged' to be tested than would have been the case under the present fully voluntary policy. Without this change of policy, it is argued that 'what once was protection of individual rights may now represent negligent practice and missed opportunities for prevention'[4]. Further, there are fears that this ultra-liberal approach to HIV has had a potentially detrimental affect on disease-control policy in general. The approach to HIV is being adopted for other diseases, so that explicit informed consent is required before tests are performed for other serious communicable diseases (such as tuberculosis) where this consent may not have previously been seen as appropriate[1]. It is claimed that while HIV policy has upheld the rights of the individual this emphasis on patient autonomy produces many missed opportunities for treatment and prevention, and it may also have created a climate in which 'we are no longer prepared to control a communicable disease epidemic' (p. 90)[2], a situation that may have disastrous consequences in light of new epidemics.

So where does this policy of focusing on individuals' autonomy leave clinical practice? It might be argued that, while autonomy should usually be respected, there are instances in clinical practice where testing *without* this 'gold standard' of voluntary fully informed consent is the right thing to do. For instance, if all patients were tested for serious communicable disease such as HIV and hepatitis before 'high-risk' procedures such as certain kinds of orthopaedic surgery, this may allow health-care workers to make a more accurate assessment of the risk involved and take appropriate measures; if all pregnant women were tested for HIV then steps could be taken to reduce the risk of perinatal transmission of the virus; if physicians could use their judgement as to which diseases a patient should be tested for without gaining explicit consent from the patient then opportunities for treatment would not be missed. As we will see, while some groups such as pregnant women *are* seen as exceptions to the rule, in all other cases that deal with competent adults, policy in this area, such as the General Medical Council (GMC) guidelines, prohibit these infringements of autonomy (however well meaning) and insist that patients need to give uncoerced and explicit consent before these tests are performed.

The General Medical Council's guidance to doctors on serious infectious diseases

In September 1997, the GMC published its guidance for doctors on *Serious Communicable Diseases*[5]. This guidance is a good example of how policy relating to communicable diseases has been influenced by the current emphasis on patient autonomy. This booklet replaced the earlier *HIV Infection and AIDS*[6], and it expands the advice on consent to testing for HIV to include testing for tuberculosis and hepatitis. This guidance defines a serious communicable disease as 'any disease which may be transmitted from human to human and which may result in death or serious illness.'[5] This in particular refers to HIV, tuberculosis and hepatitis B and C.

While the GMC guidelines deal with a number of pertinent issues relating to communicable diseases – such as discrimination, consent, confidentiality and the responsibilities of doctors who have been exposed to serious communicable diseases – the major concern of the guidance is the issue of consent. The GMC guidance stresses that fully informed consent must be gained from patients before they are tested for a serious communicable disease. The only exceptions to this standard are where the patient is under 16 years old and has not reached sufficient maturity to understand the implications of testing. In the case of children, parents may consent to testing if it is held to be in the interests of the child that they be tested. Similarly, unconscious patients may be tested without consent if such testing is deemed to be in their immediate clinical interests. In practice, this means that while the principles of necessity and best interests allow unconscious or incapacitated patients to be tested for communicable diseases without their consent, where the patient is competent and able to give consent then their uncoerced consent must be gained before testing. So, even if a surgeon is undergoing a procedure that involves a high risk of blood-to-blood contact, he or she cannot insist that this patient is tested for HIV and hepatitis, or other blood-borne diseases, before the procedure.

The guidelines do tackle the problem of testing of patients in order to assess the risk of infection for health-care workers who have suffered a needlestick injury, or other occupational exposure to blood or body fluids. But again, the guidance is that consent should be gained before testing is undertaken. In certain exceptional circumstances it may be acceptable to test without the consent of the patient: if, for instance, 'you have good reason to think that the patient may have a condition such as HIV for which prophylactic treatment is available' (paragraph 9)[5], but, in such circumstances, those requesting the test must be prepared to justify this action to the courts, their employer or the GMC.

In line with this emphasis on consent, the guidance stipulates that confidentiality may only be breached in exceptional circumstances 'in order to protect a person from death or serious harm' (paragraph 19)[5]. Where such disclosure is undertaken, the patient should be told prior to the disclosure, and those making the decision to disclose this information must be prepared to justify this decision.

As well as a duty to protect the autonomy of their patients, doctors also have a duty to protect patients against infection. Under this guidance, doctors have a duty to keep well informed about communicable diseases and to always take appropriate measures to protect themselves and their patients from infection. If a doctor has any reason to believe they have been exposed to a serious communicable disease they should seek and follow professional advice as to whether to undergo testing. However, there is no absolute duty to be tested; testing is required only where failing to be tested puts others at risk of death or serious harm. What counts as a risk of death or serious harm and who decides this, however, are not indicated. According to the guidance, doctors are entitled to the same confidentiality and support as other patients, with breaches of confidentiality only justified where there is good reason to believe that patients are at risk of infection.

The message given in these guidelines is that individual autonomy and privacy should be maintained even when dealing with serious infectious diseases. The only exceptions to this rule are either where the patient is unable to consent or where an identifiable third party is at risk of death or serious harm. Consequently, in most cases, testing for diseases such as HIV, tuberculosis and hepatitis B and C should be fully voluntary and only undertaken after informed consent for such a test is obtained.

These guidelines are in line with the 'new' climate of disease control that worries many commentators. The focus of such guidelines is on the individual rights of the infected rather than the protection of third parties, with great caution advised wherever there is a call to test either a patient or a colleague without explicit, freely given consent. Is this the most acceptable approach to serious communicable diseases, or is this an over-demanding standard that will lead to missed opportunities for individuals and lack of control of infection?

For those serious communicable diseases for which effective treatment and disease control measures exist, it might be argued that widespread screening programmes should be put in place, not only to allow treatment of those infected and prevention for those who are not but also to allay fears of infection, and the stigmatisation and discrimination that often accompany fear. For instance, routine screening of patients undergoing surgery may be justified on the grounds of protection of third parties and best interests of the patient, but only if it can be shown that these grounds justify the infringement of patient autonomy that this policy would entail. Is there a case to say that these and similar guidelines are over-demanding and that, in some cases, it is acceptable to test without explicit and freely given consent?

Informed consent an over-demanding standard?

There are those who argue that it is not appropriate to insist that testing for serious infectious diseases should be voluntary and accompanied by explicit informed consent. Gibson and Seaton from the British Thoracic Society[1] argue that the GMC's standard on consent for testing for a serious communicable disease is unnecessarily simplistic and sets an over-zealous standard. They argue that testing for tuberculosis should only require informed consent when the suspicion of tuberculosis infection is high. Gibson and Seaton suggest that where the suspicion of tuberculosis infection is low 'asking for general permission to test samples to exclude infection is appropriate without necessarily specifically naming tuberculosis when the probability of the patient having the disease is comparatively low'[1]. Their claim is that requiring the same levels of consent for tuberculosis as are required for HIV will lead to unnecessary distress for patients and many missed opportunities for treatment and prevention.

After correspondence with the British Thoracic Society, the Standards Committee of the GMC revisited this issue in response to this criticism. The committee agreed that if non-specific investigations such as a chest X-ray was undertaken, whether the patient should be told about the possibility of detecting tuberculosis should depend upon the likelihood of it being found. However, if a test is undertaken that is specifically designed to detect tuberculosis then the patient should be fully informed of this before testing occurs[7]. Thus, the overwhelming view of the Committee was that:

> . . . it was no longer acceptable to advise doctors, that, as a matter of principle, they may undertake testing for serious conditions without the patient's knowledge or agreement. . . . As in other parts of medicine, we as doctors cannot hope to maintain the trust and respect of our patients unless we share information with them, respect their right to autonomy, and treat them as partners in the decision making process.[7]

Breathnach, a consultant medical microbiologist, in response to the GMC's stance on this issue, argues that:

> The GMC guidance, if strictly enforced, would lead to an absurd and damaging situation. Chandler (on the behalf of the GMC) implies that doctors can only hold the trust of the public by adopting a servile and inefficient approach to making a diagnosis, under the guise of respecting the autonomy of patients. This is to confuse what is politically desirable with what is ethical and right. It is regrettable that the GMC cannot see the difference.[8]

Breathnach argues that:

> on receiving a sputum sample from a patient with fevers, weight loss and a chronic cough, it is standard practice to look for acid-fast bacilli, even if the clinicians have not thought of TB . In fact, we would be considered negligent if these tests were omitted. It would be foolish and impracticable to try and obtain informed consent from all such cases, yet that is what the GMC advise.[8]

He argues that the emphasis on autonomy that characterised policy relating to HIV, if applied to other areas of medical policy, while perhaps seen by many to be politically desirable, may lead to harm to patients in the form of missed diagnoses and increased risk of infection.

Is the approach advocated by the GMC the appropriate approach to serious infectious diseases? Are we justified in infringing autonomy in order to protect others from infection and, possibly, to protect the best interests of those unaware of their infection, or do all patients have a right to remain in ignorance of their health state?

Right to remain in ignorance?

There is much debate surrounding the so-called 'right to remain in ignorance' especially when it relates to information about potentially serious health conditions. On one side of the debate, it is argued that it is important that a person's decisions are as maximally autonomous as possible and that choices can only be deemed autonomous if the individual making them has all the available relevant information. As information about one's health state is important when making decisions, medical or not, there can be no right to remain in ignorance of information relating to one's own health. On the other hand, it is argued that principle of respect for individual autonomy dictates that competent individuals have the right to decline information about their health status even where this action is thought, by others, to be contrary to their best interests. Just as we allow competent individuals to make other 'risky' or perhaps ill-advised decisions about how they lead their lives, such as taking up a dangerous sport or having a very unhealthy diet, so perhaps we should allow individuals to keep their heads in the sand about their possible health states.

Whatever the truth about the debate surrounding the 'right to remain in ignorance' of one's health state, there is a strong case in arguing that the issues change dramatically when considering the related but distinct issue of whether individuals have a right to refuse tests that will provide information about not only their own health state, but also information that may allow them to protect others from harm. Even the most liberal of commentators would argue that it may be ethically justifiable to thwart an individual's autonomous choices in order to protect a third party from harm. This, of course, is the rationale behind traditional Public Health measures, which, in extreme circumstances, allow provision to detain or enforce treatment on those with dangerous infectious diseases, in order to protect the wider public from infection*. So, while an individual may, arguably, have the right to refuse information or treatment and in doing so risk his or her

---

* In the United Kingdom, for instance, the Public Health (Control of Diseases) Act 1984 empowers public health officers to act to prevent the spread of disease. The powers conferred by the Act and the Public Health (Infectious Diseases) Regulations 1988 permit the state to override virtually all individual liberties in the cause of protecting the community.

own health or happiness, it seems that if this right exists it is weakened by a risk to third parties from this decision. Consequently, it can be argued that there are justifiable exceptions to this 'right' to individual autonomy in medical decision making. The protection of the physical well-being of others and their autonomy sometimes dictates that an individual's autonomous choices may be overridden.

One good example of this is policy response to HIV in pregnant women. Since reports in 1994 suggested that maternal–foetal HIV transmission could be reduced by the use of zidovudine (ZDV)[9], there has been a general trend towards viewing pregnant women and newborns as exceptions to the usual opposition to coercive HIV testing policies. While the GMC and other regulating bodies such as the American Medical Association insist that HIV testing should, in most circumstances, be freely chosen and preceded by explicit informed consent, testing in pregnancy is seen as an exception to this rule. This approach to HIV testing in pregnancy has found its way into policy in most developed countries. For instance, the UK government implemented policy in 1999 to recommend an HIV test as part of their routine antenatal screening tests[10]. Similarly, in May 2000, the American College of Obstetricians and Gynecologists announced that every pregnant woman in the United States, regardless of her apparent risk, should be tested for HIV as a routine part of antenatal care[11].

While there have been calls to make antenatal testing for HIV mandatory[12], in the main the testing programmes that have been implemented have involved routine testing where pregnant women do have the option to refuse the test. It is, perhaps, not immediately clear that this kind of routine testing with the option of 'opting out' infringes these women's autonomy. There are, however, compelling reasons to suggest that routine testing of this kind is coercive, albeit to a lesser extent than mandatory testing. It is clear that programmes of routine testing are implemented in order to ensure that more people are tested than if the test had only been *offered*. Thus, the fundamental aim of routine testing is to secure the testing of not only those women who would have elected to be tested but also those women who would not have specifically chosen to be tested. If policy is to ensure that high levels of uptake of routine testing are achieved then it would seem that non-directive counselling will be impossible. Referring to antenatal screening programmes that involve routine testing for genetic disorders, Angus Clarke points out

> the very existence of a screening program amounts in effect to a recommendation that the testing thereby made available is a good thing. Health professionals and society would hardly establish and promote antenatal screening for Down's syndrome unless they wanted people to make use of it – the existence of such a programme is an implicit, but powerful, recommendation to accept any screening offer made. Screening programs therefore, simply cannot be non-directive. Health professionals may respect the decisions of those who decline the offer of screening, not coercing them into compliance, but those who decide against participation will carry a label of social deviance unless great efforts have been made to avoid this. In practice, at least some of the personnel offering such tests are likely to regard those

who decline screening as irritating, if not irresponsible, and to make this clear to their 'clients'. (p. 401)[13]

Where routine testing programmes aim to achieve 90% uptake (p. 2)[10] or even 'make HIV testing as commonplace as urinalysis during the first prenatal office visit'[14] such programmes will necessarily contain some degree of coercion.

However, even if it is accepted that routine antenatal HIV testing involves a degree of coercion that would be deemed unacceptable in other circumstances, this does not necessarily mean that such testing is unacceptable. While such coercion may not be justifiable on the paternalistic grounds that the individual should have this information for her own benefit, it may be justifiable to avoid harm to her future child. As has already been discussed, it can be ethically justifiable to use coercion if by doing so a third party is protected. This is the basis on which mandatory treatment of infectious diseases was traditionally implemented, and it is the rationale behind the implementation of routine antenatal testing regimens. By increasing the uptake of testing, it is hoped that harm to future children will be avoided. But are future children protected from harm by these tests and, if so, does this justify the infringement of pregnant women's autonomy?

Protection from harm

There are compelling arguments to support the claim that routine HIV testing in pregnancy is justifiable, even if it involves a degree of coercion. There is evidence that identifying HIV infection in pregnancy may help to protect future children from HIV infection. Early indications were that women who are diagnosed as HIV positive in pregnancy may reduce the risk of passing the infection on to their child from around 25% to around 8% by using zidovudine during pregnancy, giving birth by caesarian section and avoiding breast-feeding[15]. More recent preliminary data indicate that the use of these risk-reducing measures may lower the risk of perinatal transmission to around 2%[16]. While it might be argued that most individuals have a right to remain in ignorance of their HIV status in normal circumstances, there seem to be good reasons to suppose that pregnant women, on the strength of the available evidence, may have a moral duty to be tested for HIV in order to attempt to prevent their child from being infected with the virus.

While routine testing of pregnant women might be morally acceptable, what is not clear is that routine testing is the preferable course of action (we will return to this point later), or that pregnant women alone are an exceptional case where testing for serious disease can be undertaken without the usual requirement for non-coercive fully informed consent. If it is justifiable to infringe a pregnant woman's autonomy in order to attempt to protect a third party (her future child) then why is it not justifiable to implement similarly autonomy-limiting policies in order to protect the contacts of individuals with serious infectious diseases from infection?

Is it possible that the sort of 'covert' testing advocated by Gibson and Seaton[1] and Breathnach[8] could be justified on similar grounds, or even the routine testing of all patients attending medical institutions or all health-care workers?

Protection of others: health-care workers and patients

Between July 1997 and June 2000, surveillance of occupational exposure to blood-borne viruses was undertaken in the UK. Occupational health departments were requested to submit data outlining the circumstances of any work-related exposure to infection from patients who were known to be infected with HIV, hepatitis C or hepatitis B. A total of 813 reports were received. The most commonly exposed groups were nurses and midwives (45%) and doctors (38%), and percutaneous injuries (needlestick or sharps cut) were the most commonly reported type of exposure (70%). Among the 293 exposures to HIV, there was one confirmed transmission of the disease and none among the 462 exposures to hepatitis C. This case of HIV transmission brings the total number of occupationally acquired HIV infections reported in the UK to five, with a further 11 cases involving health-care workers working overseas in areas of high prevalence[17].

While the risk of infection from patient to health-care worker is low (around 3% transmission rate from a source infected with hepatitis C and 0.03% for a single percutaneous exposure to HIV infected blood[18]) anxiety surrounding such instances of exposure remain understandably high. This anxiety is further understandable when one considers that a high proportion of those infected with HIV and hepatitis remain undiagnosed. For instance, in the UK in 1999, 52% of the heterosexual men found to be HIV positive by unlinked anonymous surveillance at Genito-urinary Medicine clinics were undiagnosed, with 42% of HIV-positive women and 37% of HIV-positive homosexual and bisexual men surveyed also undiagnosed[19]. While health-care workers can protect their contacts and make use of any prophylactic treatment available if they are aware of their patient's infection, this would not be possible with undiagnosed infections. While there is provision to test patients without their consent for serious infectious diseases[5], those undertaking such testing must suspect infection and be prepared to justify their actions. Furthermore, while the use of 'universal precautions' is recommended during all potentially risky contact with patients[20], anecdotal evidence suggests that most surgeons only use such measures if the patient is known to be infected. A recent study in Leeds showed that, out of all 260 patients with HIV infection, 24 patients underwent a total of 28 operations under general anaesthesia when their HIV status was as yet undiagnosed[21].

On the other side of the equation, there have been at least 12 clusters of hepatitis B infections in the United Kingdom where infected health-care workers are thought to be the source of infection[22]. The risk of health-care workers infecting a patient with hepatitis or HIV is much lower than the risk of them being infected by patients[23]. It has been estimated that the risk of transmission of HIV from an infected health-care worker to a patient is between 1 in 4000 and 1 in 40000[24]. The risk of HIV infection from a health-care worker is thought to be 100 times less than the risk of hepatitis B infection[25]. Only two cases of HIV transmission from infected health-care workers have been reported[26,27]. But while the risk of HIV is relatively low, it has been suggested that the *overall* risk to patients is similar to hepatitis B, as HIV carries a 100 times greater risk of death than does hepatitis B[25].

214

At present, there is no widespread screening of health-care workers for serious communicable diseases in the UK. Testing of health-care workers is on a voluntary basis, but those who are known to be infected with HIV or hepatitis B may not undertake exposure-prone procedures[28,29]. However, three cases of HIV-infected doctors, in Glasgow in the early 1990s, illustrate the limitations of this advice. All three doctors were only diagnosed as being HIV positive after they developed late HIV-related diseases[30]. If it is felt important that infected health-care workers should not undertake exposure-prone procedures, and if voluntary testing and disclosure is not achieving this aim, then there seems to be a case for the compulsory or routine testing of health-care workers for serious communicable diseases.

If infringing the autonomy of pregnant women is deemed acceptable, as it provides information useful to the women about their infection and facilitates the protection of third parties, then couldn't the same grounds be used to justify the routine testing of all patients, or perhaps all patients undergoing invasive treatment, and even the routine testing of health-care workers involved in exposure-prone procedures?

There would clearly be problems with such widespread screening of patients and health-care workers. Such a programme would be costly to implement, may cause anxiety in those being tested and may be impractical and difficult to implement, but these are all problems that apply equally to the programme of routine antenatal HIV testing. It may also be claimed that the risk of infection from health-care worker to patient or vice versa is so low as not to justify such a widespread screening policy but, again, a similar point can be made about the routine testing of pregnant women. While the UK policy of routine antenatal HIV testing is applied nationwide, the incidence of HIV outside London and a few other urban areas is so low that many antenatal clinics are likely never to treat an HIV-positive pregnant woman. It might also be argued that it is possible for patients and their carers to be protected from communicable disease infection without necessarily being tested for these diseases. It would be difficult, and perhaps unwise, for a pregnant women to undertake the therapeutic interventions that may protect her child from being infected with HIV without knowing that she was in fact HIV positive. Health-care workers can protect their patients and be protected from their patients by employing 'universal precautions' at all times. However, 'universal precautions' sometimes fail and, in such cases, a positive diagnosis of infection may be necessary in order to implement prophylactic treatment and protection of sexual contacts.

Conclusions

The policy of routine antenatal HIV testing stands out amongst the current approaches to HIV and other serious communicable diseases that place great emphasis on individual autonomy and informed consent. There are calls to extend this approach from pregnant women to other areas of disease-control policy, either in the guise of routine testing of other groups, such as patients and health-care workers engaged in exposure-prone procedures, or the covert testing of patients either in their 'best interests' or in order to establish risk in cases of accidental exposure. What direction is taken will depend on the importance that is placed on the principle of individual autonomy. If it is felt that individual autonomy is so important that, in all but very extreme cases, it outweighs any benefits that might be gained by infringing it then these calls for non-voluntary testing must be abandoned. If it is felt that giving people information that may allow them to make better decisions about their health and the health of those around them is worth infringing autonomy in this way then policies must be developed that allow this provision but limit it only to cases where this justification applies. Whatever is decided, it is important that the same rule is applied across the board. If infringing the autonomy of health-care professionals is not deemed justifiable, even in order to possibly benefit themselves and their patients, then infringing the autonomy of pregnant women on the same grounds cannot be justifiable either. While there may be good practical and moral reasons why pregnant women should be tested for HIV this does not necessarily mean that routine testing should be the preferred option, especially where comparable groups are not subjected to the same degree of coercion.

References

1. Gibson GJ, Seaton A. GMC's advice in Serious Communicable Diseases. Br Med J 2000; 320: 1727
2. Richards EP III. HIV Testing, Screening, and Confidentiality: An American Perspective. In: HIV and AIDS: Testing, Screening and Confidentiality. R Bennett, CA Erin, eds. Oxford: Oxford University Press, 1999: 75–90
3. Bayer R. Public Health Policy and the AIDS epidemic. An End to AIDS Exceptionalism? N Engl J Med 1991; 324: 1500–4
4. De Cock KM, Johnson AM. From exceptionalism to normalisation: a reappraisal of attitudes and practice around HIV testing. Br Med J 1998; 316: 290–3
5. General Medical Council. Serious Communicable Diseases. GMC, 1997 [published on the internet at: http://www.gmc-uk.org/standards/standards_frameset.htm]
6. General Medical Council. HIV Infection and AIDS. London: GMC, 1993
7. Chantler C. A reply to GJ Gibson et al GMC's advice on Serious Communicable Diseases. Br Med J 2000; 320: 1727
8. Breathnach AS. Consent to testing for tuberculosis [an electronic response to GJ Gibson and A Seaton. GMC's advice on Serious Communicable Diseases. Br Med J 2000; 320: 1727] published on the internet at http://www.bmj.com/cgi/eletters/320/7251/1727]
9. Connor EM, Sperling MD, Gelber R, et al. The Pediatric AIDS Clinical Trials Group, Reduction of maternal–infant transmission of human immunodeficiency virus type 1 with AZT treatment. N Engl J Med 1994; 311: 1173–80
10. NHS Executive. Reducing mother to baby transmission of HIV. Health Service Circular [HSC 1999/183]. London: NHS Executive, 1999
11. American College of Obstetricians and Gynecologists. News release: HIV tests urged for all pregnant women: Ob-Gyn launch campaign for universal HIV screening. Published online by the American College of Obstetriticians and Gynecologists, May 23 2000. http://www.acog.org/from_home/publications/press_releases/nr 05-23-00-2.cfm
12. Rovner J. US specialists object to AMA's call for mandatory testing. Lancet 1996; 348: 330
13. Clarke A. Genetic Counselling. In: Encyclopaedia of Applied Ethics, Vol. 2. R. Chadwick, ed. San Diego: Academic Press, 1998: 391–405
14. Greene MF. Chair of the American Association of Obstetricians and Gynecologists Committee on Obstetric Practice reported by the American Medical Association. 2000 at: http://www.ama-assn.org/ama/pub/article/1987–2565.html

15. Centres for Disease Control. AZT for the prevention of HIV transmission from mother to infant. Morb Mortal Wkly Rep 1994; 43: 285–7

16. Mofenson LM. Technical report: perinatal human immunodeficiency virus testing and prevention of transmission. Commission on Pediatric AIDS [Review]. Pediatrics 2000; 106: E88

17. Evans B, Duggan W, Baker J, Ramsay M, Abiteboul D. Exposure of healthcare workers in England, Wales and Northern Ireland to bloodborne viruses between July 1997 and June 2000: analysis of surveillance data. Br Med J 2001; 322: 397–8

18. Scottish Executive. Needlestick injuries: sharpen your awareness. 2002. Published on the internet at: *http://www.scotland.gov.uk/ library3/health/nisa–06.asp*

19. Unlinked Anonymous Surveys Steering Group. Department of Health Prevalence of HIV and hepatitis infections in the United Kingdom 1999. London: Department of Health, 2000

20. Advisory Committee on Dangerous Pathogens. Protection against blood-borne infections in the workplace: HIV and hepatitis. London: HMSO, 1995

21. Walker PP, Reynolds MT. Universal Precautions should be used during all surgical procedures. [Letter]. Br Med J 1998; 316: 701

22. Heptonstall J. Outbreaks of hepatitis B virus infection associated with infected surgical staff. Communicable Disease Report Weekly 1991; 8: R81–4

23. Heptonstall J, Porter K, Gill ON. Occupational transmission of HIV – summary of published reports. London: Communicable Diseases Surveillance Centre, 1995

24. Bell DM, Martone WJ, Culver DH, et al. Risk of endemic HIV and hepatitis B virus transmission to patients during invasive procedures. Abstracts of VII International Conference on AIDS. Florence: Intituto Superiore di Sanita, 1991

25. Webber DJ, Hoffmann KK, Kutala WA. Management of the health care worker infected with human immunodeficiency virus: lessons from nosocomial transmission of hepatitis B virus. Infect Control Hospital Epidemiol 1991; 12: 625–30

26. Anonymous. Transmission of HIV from an infected surgeon to a patient in France. Communicable Disease Report Weekly 1997; 7: 17

27. Anonymous. Possible transmission of human immunodeficiency virus to a patient during an invasive dental procedure. Morbidity Mortality Weekly Report 1990; 39: 489–93

28. The United Kingdom Advisory Group on Hepatitis. Protecting health care workers and patients from hepatitis B. London: HMSO Health Publications Unit, 1993

29. UK Departments of Health. AIDS-HIV infected health care workers: guidance on the management of infected health care workers. Edinburgh: Scottish Office Home and Health Department, 1993

30. Pell J, Gruer L, Christie P, Goldberg D. Management of HIV infected health care workers; lessons from three cases. Br Med J 1996; 312: 1150–2

217

Teaching and Assessing Medical Ethics 16

Lisa Schwartz

Introduction

Becoming a doctor bestows certain privileges. With privilege comes accountability, which cannot be responsibly undertaken without knowledge and clinical skills. Medical accountability must also include the ability to manage the uncertainty inherent in helping fellow human beings while remaining consistent with a consensus on professional limitations. These limitations include laws, skills, knowledge and economics, as well as a duty to expand the boundaries that will enhance patient care. Learning ethics and law as they are relevant to the medical context will enable physicians to enact their duties responsibly and even question those duties where the needs of particular individuals require it.

The aims of teaching medical ethics

The emphasis and commitment that health-care ethics has received from professional organisations leave little room to doubt that the governing bodies commend the teaching of medical ethics and law in medical schools. The endorsements in statements, such as that made in *Tomorrow's Doctors*[1] and similar ones expressed about the educational requirements for all health professionals, demonstrate firm commitments to the teaching of ethics.

If the presumption is that medical ethics ought to be taught then it is worth considering what we hope to achieve by teaching ethics to medical students. In teaching ethics, do we hope to produce doctors who know and follow the ethical and legal requirements of the profession as these are expressed in professional consensus statements and in law, or do we want doctors who are capable of critically assessing a given ethical problem and, in the light of general moral principles, deciding what is the best way of proceeding, *even if* it is in opposition to professional consensus and legal statutes? In simpler terms, do we want doctors who know the law and obey it, or do we want doctors who can think about what is best to do and base a decision on the features of a case? Do we want medical lawyers or medical philosophers?

The dichotomy may be uncomfortable, but it simplifies the ideas and conforms to prejudices about what teaching ethics can do for medical practitioners. Ideally, we will be able to find a middle ground that is less compromise and more an image of responsible practitioners who understand their obligations and apply them conscientiously.

The stated aims of programmes in medical ethics and law tend to vary in medical schools, but there is likely to be more intended agreement than disagreement regarding what we hope to achieve with such courses. The potential for agreement is embodied in the General Medical Council (GMC) aims for medical education expressed in *Tomorrow's Doctors*[1], which states that all graduating medical students must be able to demonstrate:

> awareness of the moral and ethical responsibilities involved in individual patient care and in the provision of care to populations of patients; such awareness must be developed early in the course

This is a broad but worthy remit. The field is permeated with such commendable statements 'to improve patient care', or 'to develop practitioners with the ability to apply their skills critically and with wisdom' and, more modestly, 'to inform potential practitioners of their legal duties and professional responsibilities'. In the end we are left with a problem. The problem is one of translating the experiences gained by participating in ethics education into practical skills that are helpful in the clinical context. It is incumbent on medical schools that they provide students with suitable knowledge and skills, but that they also learn that practising ethically includes certain attitudes valued by the profession.

Is it better to have competent doctors or ethical doctors?

So far we have stated three possible models for the outcome of a professional ethics programme in medicine. These are:

- a doctor who knows and obeys the law
- a doctor who applies analytic skills or moral reasoning and adjusts decisions accordingly
- a responsible physician who knows why it is important to adhere to laws but applies them critically.

Usually, the division happens somewhat differently; the expected division is between a doctor who is competent and one who is ethical. This has become a cliché of the profession and indicates a lack of understanding. What is a competent doctor if not one who behaves ethically? Can the two really be separated in this way?

Arguments that suggest ethics and clinical competence can be separated usually claim there is no room for studying something as rarefied as ethics in a practical course. They see no relevance in considering right from wrong when such things are *common sense* and essentially irrelevant when good clinical skills are all that matter. Why study medical ethics? Why study any ethics at all, when the answers, according to this moral realist perspective, are all self-evident? Doctors, they will argue, require no training in ethics because these issues can be easily resolved by reference to the foundations for moral reasoning each of us already possesses. According to this model, regulations provide useful assistance for misguided or inexperienced practitioners, but it would be sufficient to instruct doctors of their requirements by rote and certainly unnecessary to spend valuable time debating them.

It is hard to see how this can be the case when malpractice litigation is on the rise, such as for the unauthorised retention of organs at post-mortem, and the public hotly debates medical interventions such as the separation of conjoined twins.

In response to the realist position, when it comes down to it, there is insufficient agreement about the basis of moral truths. Rather, there is a very real possibility of moral relativism, especially in free pluralistic societies that stress tolerance over enforced agreement. All of this is enough to dismiss as overly simplistic beliefs in the consistency of common sense. For example, one medical student will believe that abortion should be available to any woman who requests it, others will believe that abortion is wrong in all circumstances. Even more complicated, are the multitude of positions in between. Some believe abortion is morally acceptable under certain conditions, such as danger to the physical or psychological health of the mother. Others believe abortion is never morally right, but that it may be the lesser of two moral wrongs in some cases. The permutations are innumerable, and they illustrate how complicated and uncertain moral reasoning can become.

The analytic approach

Alternatively, students could learn that it isn't enough to simply follow professional consensus. In order to be truly responsible moral actors they must understand the reasons for the consensus. Doctors should also be able to take a contrary position when they feel it is morally required, and justify their decision. This entails developing an ability to consider contrary and opposing attitudes and to develop arguments in support of morally acceptable alternatives. The teachers of medical ethics and law in UK medical schools reinforce this in their Consensus statement published in 1998[2], which recommends:

- ensuring that students understand the ethical principles and values which underpin the practice of good medicine
- enabling students to think critically about ethical issues in medicine, to reflect upon their own beliefs about ethics, to understand and appreciate alternative and sometimes competing approaches and to be able to argue and counter-argue in order to contribute to informed discussion and debate
- enabling students not only to enjoy the intellectual satisfaction of debates within medical ethics and law but also to appreciate that ethical and legal reasoning and critical reflection are natural and integral components in their clinical decision making and practice.

This endorses an analytic approach to medical ethics that encourages students to recognise that their own beliefs may be a matter of personal judgement or taste and that these moral beliefs need to be critically reflected upon. This will improve their ability to appreciate the divergent attitudes of their colleagues, patients and professional bodies and help individual students to either build suitably convincing justifications for their own moral judgements or adjust them after reflection upon persuasive argument.

Moreover, the analytic approach encourages the freedom and capacity to challenge the status quo, without which it is widely recognised that consensus becomes dogma, and ethical practice cannot keep pace with scientific and medical progress. Students are, therefore, encouraged to learn to critically reflect on their responsibilities as professional bodies set them out, and on legal statutes, in order to ensure the justifications continue to evolve.

Finally, critical reflection or analysis of the institutional duties of a doctor permits students to assess whether the general principles that these duties are founded on apply in individual cases, or may have grown outdated and irrelevant or, potentially, violate the rights of patients and communities. For example, unconsented internal examination of unconscious patients is being reconsidered as a teaching practice[3]. It may be one aim of teaching medical ethics that students learn how to critically accept or reject the laws, codes and duties that will guide their actions as practitioners. This attitude implies that rules are open to question, and reducible to mere starting points for debate. The advantages to this perspective are flexibility and sensitivity to the differences that make each case unique, requiring context-sensitive responses. This is intended to help doctors deal with uncertainty by conforming to legal and professional expectations or rejecting them when the situation requires.

Problems with the analytic approach

This moral relativist position has significant problems of its own. First, it requires practitioners to remain open and non-judgemental of any moral difference they encounter. This is laudable for its tolerance and flexibility, but it may require doctors to accept decisions they may find morally uncomfortable or worse, for example, euthanasia or clitoridectomy (female circumcision). Second, the openness of this position will require all actors to take the time to reflect upon their decisions before they are made, paying careful attention to the views of others. This again has many salutary features, but stopping to think about why one holds certain moral beliefs can cause decision paralysis. It is for this reason that the analytic approach to medical ethics is so often criticised. There is a real danger in providing students with reasoning skills and requiring them to be sensitive to other perspectives to the extent that it hinders their ability to make decisions with any confidence. So, we expect the sensitivity of a moral relativist, who recognises the value in varying opinions and rationales, and, then again, we also hope for practitioners who can make decisions, often at a moment's notice and in the midst of crisis.

What is more, practitioners must know the consequences of breaching legal or professional obligations. If analytic medical ethics emphasises skills that encourage doctors to act contrary to professional consensus, the consequences can be perilous for them and patients. There is a danger of practitioners not fully understanding they could be held criminally accountable for an act of moral defiance that may not have been worthwhile or morally justifiable.

The teachers of medical ethics and law in UK medical schools consensus statement places equal emphasis on students learning their legal responsibilities as doctors[2]. They recommend:

- ensuring that students know the main professional obligations of doctors in the United Kingdom as endorsed by the institutions which regulate or influence medical practice particularly those specified by the General Medical Council
- giving students a knowledge and understanding of the legal process and the legal obligations of medical practitioners sufficient to enable them to practise medicine effectively and with minimal risk.

Therefore, students of medical ethics ought to be taught to do their duty as regulatory bodies and legal authorities define it. To do so acknowledges the degree of effort and experience that is applied to making these decisions in the first place. But this must be balanced with the highly valuable skills of critical argument, justification and the attitudes of openness, reflection and flexibility inherent in the analytic approach.

A combination of the two approaches is the ideal. Doctors should know and follow rules because they have been carefully decided by experienced practitioners in response to social expectations. But they must also be sensitive to moral diversity and have the integrity to challenge laws and rules if a situation of uncertainty calls for it – though they must not do so lightly!

Getting it right and getting it wrong (*or* What counts as a wrong answer on an examination?)

Without assessment, it is impossible to ensure students have truly understood the material and can actually apply it to clinical cases, even hypothetical ones. Criteria for marking presuppose the possibility of students getting it wrong. Getting it right and getting it wrong will obviously have to reflect what students are taught, and how they are taught. In the case of medical ethics and law, there may be two broad sorts of assessment. First, there is the measure of factual knowledge about laws and regulations. Then, there are more uncertain elements, such as analytic skills and ability to apply theoretical concepts to specific situations.

The first set admits greater certainty, and it can be tested by multiple choice or true/false questions. This will include assessment of students' knowledge of legal and professional expectations. How much knowledge of legal statutes a student or practitioner ought to know is debatable but, clearly, there are some statutes and guidelines that every medical practitioner should know to ensure they work within legal and professional limits. For example, all UK physicians must know their duty to refer a woman to someone who can help her obtain an abortion, and the restrictions that apply under the Abortion Act 1967. Also, every doctor should know whether assisting suicide is illegal in the country or state in which they practise.

How much jurisprudence should be taught is up to the discretion of course leaders. However, deeper understanding helps practitioners cope with the uncertainty of applying laws and rules in ambiguous situations, such as what constitutes an acceptable reason for offering an abortion or breaching confidentiality? Thus, some knowledge of the reasoning that underpins statutory judgements will help students recognise the significance of their obligations and encourage compliance.

There is some debate over whether students ought to be offered philosophical theory that may be applied to medical contexts. Many medical practitioners ask to be taught theory, so a demand exists. Some theory can be useful, such as learning to compare consequentialist or outcome oriented thinking against deontological approaches where the intention is to fulfil certain moral duties. This can help develop analytic skills that support ethical reasoning in situations where there is no consensus.

It is possible to assess theoretical material by determining whether a student has a correct understanding of a concept such as paternalism. Students can be examined for knowledge of concepts that are commonly referred to in medical journals including autonomy, beneficence and so forth. In addition, students should be able to apply theories and concepts to particular cases. Case discussion is the preferred teaching method for medical ethics because it permits students to explore their own reasoning and that of others, as well as situating the issues in context[4]. What cannot be assessed are students' attitudes because these are variable and require knowledge of intention and psychological states not accessible though examinations. However, it is possible to assess behaviour, which may reflect attitudes. Practical tests such as OSCEs, portfolio cases and modified essay questions (MEQs) are an excellent method of assessing students' understanding and abilities in ethical reasoning. In this situation, students can demonstrate 'getting it right' not simply by coming up with consensus answers, but also by demonstrating clarity of argument, balance, justification and an ability to anticipate the costs and benefits of the resolutions they propose.

Students can be coached to learn to perform all of these tasks by giving them time to discuss issues and concepts with case illustrations. Getting it right, therefore, will mean being able both to (a) identify professional consensus positions in laws and codes; and (b) apply these; and, using theoretical concepts, justify support or divergence from the consensus in hypothetical situations.

What significance should be placed on the teaching of medical ethics relative to other disciplines?

Ethics should be given sufficient weight and presence in the curriculum to ensure that it is taken seriously by all prospective practitioners. These are people who will look after us in our most vulnerable times, people to whom we will entrust the care of our children. Students need to know their legal and professional obligations in order to become responsible practitioners. This is just as important as knowing how to administer a vital injection or recognise the signs of heart attack. It is the duty of medical educators, as they are empowered by professional bodies, to ensure that doctors are safe, responsible, respectful and will not easily transgress legal or professional boundaries, either through ignorance or because of poor training.

Regular case discussions should take place throughout the entire medical school programme. These must be led by practitioners or others who understand the importance of the material and have a good grasp of the theoretical underpinnings of medical ethics. Professional ethicists have a role to play in this setting by providing a lay perspective not necessarily bound by a medical vision or by health-care professionals' loyalties. The medical perspective is valuable and professional loyalties are laudable, but they may not harmonise with social perceptions, such as the belief in personal autonomy, that have led to current approaches in medical ethics. Moreover, if the medical ethicist has a background in philosophy, theology or some other relevant field, they bring with them knowledge of the complex history of ethical theory that may not be at the fingertips of most medical practitioners.

There is scope for using lectures to inform students in a cost-effective manner but not to the exclusion of case discussion in small groups. Opportunistic teaching in wards and surgeries is an invaluable means of contextual learning. Deans, professors and professional colleagues must demonstrate their support of this material, not only as educators but also as potential role models who apply the principles of medical ethics in daily practice.

How can ethics be taught at the bedside, or in busy units like ICUs?

Early years of medical education ought to include special sessions devoted to discussion of ethics and law in medicine. These can be based around fictional cases, actual cases drawn from tutors' experiences and suitably anonymised or from the media. Cases should range from extreme and ground-breaking, such as euthanasia and stem cell research, to more mundane issues like prescribing antibiotics for sore throat or writing sick notes. Other topics ought to cover micro issues, such as doctor–patient relationship; and macro issues like allocation of resources. Early years are a good time to lay the foundations of analytic skills and ethical theories that can help facilitate ethical decision making as well as encourage students to learn professional and legal duties of a doctor.

Ethics training must continue in the clinical years. Otherwise, studies indicate that students loose their sensitivity to ethical issues and neglect ethical reasoning in clinical situations[5,6]. In the clinical years, ethics should be demonstrated to be a relevant part of ordinary practice as well as discussed in significant incident analyses and informal or grand rounds.

The spectre of the hidden curriculum haunts all medical education. It is understood to be the unwritten and unacknowledged aspect of the course that presents students with examples of good and bad practice on which to base their own approaches. Every practitioner has anecdotal lessons from encounters with best and worst examples of professional behaviour. These examples prove to be more

225

memorable than intended. This places a significant burden upon clinical educators to be aware of their practices and how they behave toward patients, colleagues and students.

This raises the very real concern that students will witness unethical practice and negligence by senior colleagues and teachers[7]. An atmosphere of reflective practice would deal constructively with most cases. Students could be given the opportunity to explore the event and recognise the values being applied and their appropriateness in the context. In more serious situations, where it is warranted, students must have a mechanism for taking their concerns to an academic advisor so the issue can be dealt with in accordance with institutional policy. In no way should clinically based ethics teaching become a mechanism for policing practice, nor should students be put in positions of having to defend ethical stances against bullying tutors or peer pressure.

It is crucial that students also learn responsible ways of whistle blowing if it becomes necessary. Professional organisations have recently recommended whistle blowing on colleagues for significant reasons, but they have not approached the notion with a view of the history and theory that permeates business ethics and political theory[8]. This is an area that requires development to ensure students are aware of the potential dangers inherent in whistle blowing.

The effects of the hidden curriculum can be constructive if clinical teachers are willing to model exemplary conduct. No one expects clinical tutors to be perfect in every way. Sometimes, it is the acknowledgement of frailties, or the willingness to accept imperfections and improve upon them, that make the best learning opportunities. Educational theorists recommend reflective practice and conscientious application of ethical procedures as just two ways of helping students learn by positive illustration[9,10]. For example, exhibiting respectful treatment of patients by confirming with the patient, while students are present, the patients' willingness to participate in teaching. Tutors might demonstrate reflective practice by taking a moment to explain to a student the reasons for a given clinical decision and permitting the student to ask questions and explore the choices made.

What ethics should be taught in a multicultural society?

A multicultural approach is essential in contemporary medical ethics. Presumed secularism is, mostly, disguised western practices that have dominated bioethics and represent only a single cultural perspective. All health-care practitioners must be prepared to encounter and work within a variety of cultures and social expectations. For example, western bioethics prizes respect for patient autonomy, which characterises patient-centred care. However, not all cultures see autonomy as the core governing principle of ethical practice. Japanese and Samoan traditions, for example, favour beneficence over autonomy and advocate paternalism more readily than western medical ethics does. Doctors must be prepared to function within these expectations with a non-prejudicial perspective.

Preparation for ethical practice in a multicultural setting requires the skills inherent in the analytic approach to ethics. Critical openness to other perspectives, critical self-reflection, debate and justification all need to be employed to ensure doctors act respectfully towards difference while recognising their own integrity and that of the profession.

Conclusion

This chapter has not sought to establish a list of topics that should be taught in medical ethics courses. That has been done successfully in the consensus statement already mentioned[2], and it is an ongoing project in response to social and medical developments. Rather, it seeks to explore process instead of content, and makes a case for teaching and assessing medical ethics and law in an effort to produce responsible and functioning doctors. This involves teaching and assessing students to ensure they know the legal and professional boundaries that apply to them as medical students and doctors.

Appropriate medical ethics education includes teaching and assessing students' knowledge of laws and codes. It also requires that students learn analytic skills and theory in order to comply with their duties responsibly and, if necessary, reject professional consensus in a safe and competent manner. Doctors are in privileged positions of authority and must help patients negotiate complicated health-care systems to ensure the best possible outcome. To do so they need to be able to apply ethical reasoning in situations of uncertainty and understand the law as it applies to them.

References

1. General Medical Council. Tomorrow's Doctors. London: General Medical Council, 1993
2. Doyle L, Gillon R. Consensus statement of teachers of medical ethics and law in UK medical schools. J Med Ethics 1998; 24: 188–92
3. Coldicott Y, Roberts CJC. Is current practice in the teaching of intimate examinations good enough? Ethical issues raised by a survey of students at a medical school in the UK. Presented at ASME Annual Scientific Meeting, 2001
4. Goldie J. Review of ethics curricula in undergraduate medical education. Med Edu 2000; 34: 108–19
5. Self DJ, Wolinsky FD, Baldwin DC. The effects of teaching medical ethics on medical students' moral reasoning. Acad Med 1989; 64: 755–9
6. Hebert PC, Meslin EM, Dunn EV. Measuring the ethical sensitivity of medical students: a study at the University of Toronto. J Med Ethics 1992; 18: 142–7
7. Hicks L, Lin Y, Robertson DW, et al. Understanding the clinical dilemmas that shape medical students' ethical development: questionnaire survey and focus group study. Br Med J 2001; 322: 709–10
8. Callahan JC. Ethical Issues in Professional Life. Oxford: Oxford University Press, 1988
9. Christakis DA, Feudtner C. Making the rounds: The ethical development of medical students in the context of clinical rotations. Hastings Centre Report 1994; 24: 6–12
10. Conroy SA. Professional Craft Knowledge and curricula: What are we really teaching? In: Practice Knowledge and Expertise in the Health Professions. J Higgs, A. Titchen, eds. Location: Butterworth-Heinemann, 2000

Ethical Issues in Private Practice   17

Chris Barham

Introduction

One of the advantages of working for a large monopoly employer, such as the National Health Service (NHS), should be that it provides an umbrella and a framework for identifying ethical, moral and legal issues in medical practice. Whilst this has not prevented difficulties arising in the past, it is clear that working in the independent sector requires a greater degree of individual responsibility and, therefore, may leave one more exposed[1].

It is naturally fundamental that the ethical values on which treatment of private patients are based should be the same as those for all patients, but there will, nevertheless, be special requirements related to, for example, legal, contractual and financial matters. In the UK, where the NHS provides free health-care at the point of delivery, private health-care can be taken to mean all services provided outside the NHS. This used to be a fairly clear distinction and, even when private facilities were available within the NHS, patients using them were being treated under private contract and not as part of their NHS entitlement.

In recent years, however, the distinction has become more blurred. Although the number of private patients treated in NHS hospitals has declined, other scenarios have arisen. NHS patients may be treated in private hospitals under waiting list or other initiatives which may, in some cases, mean treating them on a fee basis and in others as part of one's NHS duties. More recently, the NHS has taken new steps along this path, for example, purchasing a private hospital for combined NHS and private use, contracting with independent providers for the use of the entire facilities and staff of another, and offering patients the opportunity for private treatment when it is not available promptly within the NHS. At the time of writing, however, the principles of the NHS (that it should be free at the point of use and based on clinical need rather than the ability to pay) have been restated, although there is considerable debate about the most effective method of funding.

Despite the increased lack of clarity, it can be assumed that private practice will include any work that is done on a self-employed basis, as opposed to work as a salaried employee (usually of the NHS). In the former role, one is working as an independently contracted professional and, in doing so, taking on many of the responsibilities of the employer. The primary motive for undertaking private practice is usually financial, and there is nothing wrong with that, any more than taking on additional work as part of salaried employment. There are other motives, however, including the ability to have greater control over one's work, and being able to work in different environments.

Weller, writing on private practice, made three caveats to his paper: that it referred to private medicine as practised in the UK, that it applied mainly to provision of anaesthetic services rather than critical care and chronic pain, and that it was a personal opinion[2]. These caveats are also true for this paper, but the reason for the last – that there were no written instructions or defined rules – is no longer the case. In recent years, largely as a result of a number of high profile cases of misconduct in the independent sector, an increasing quantity of legislation and professional guidelines have been produced, which will be explored here. Indeed, we are constantly reminded of our responsibilities from many sources, including the Government, the General Medical Council (GMC), insurers and the private hospitals.

Duties of a doctor

The duties and responsibilities of doctors have been described by the GMC in their booklet Good Medical Practice[3]. These are summarised in Box 1, and they are as applicable in private health-care as they are in any other system.

Box 1: Duties of a Doctor
• make the care of your patient your first concern
• treat every patient politely and considerately
• respect patients' dignity and privacy
• listen to patients and respect their views
• give patients information in a way they can understand
• respect the rights of patients to be fully involved in decisions about their care
• keep your professional knowledge and skills up to date
• recognise the limits of your professional competence
• be honest and trustworthy
• respect and protect confidential information
• make sure that your personal beliefs do not prejudice your patients' care
• act quickly to protect patients from risk if you have good reason to believe that you or a colleague may not be fit to practise
• avoid abusing your position as a doctor
• work with colleagues in the ways that best serve patients' interests.

There is also some particular advice on financial and commercial dealings, some of which require further consideration:

You should provide information about fees and charges before obtaining patients' consent to treatment wherever possible.

This very sensible statement can present difficulties to the anaesthetist, especially when the first point of contact is immediately prior to surgery. It can, quite reasonably, be argued that this is not the time to start discussing financial matters and that the proper time is when admission is being arranged. When working as a regular team, good communication between surgeon, anaesthetist and their respective secretaries can ensure that the patient receives this information at the right time, but there are many situations in which this is not possible. Although the words 'wherever possible' are included in this particular guidance, it remains to be seen how this is viewed in practice. The establishment of a group practice may be beneficial in this respect, and this will be considered later in this chapter.

The GMC continues:

You must not exploit patients' vulnerability or lack of medical knowledge when making charges for treatment or services.

Sometimes there is the impression that some anaesthetists (and surgeons) may be a little creative in describing (and coding) the procedure in order to maximise the benefit payable. The procedure schedules produced by the insurance companies do not help this by having vague definitions (what is the difference between an 'excision' and a 'wide excision'?). However, flagrant transgressions of this principle are, at least, unethical and, at worst, fraudulent.

Moreover:

You must not put pressure on patients to accept private treatment.

Usually, this is not an issue for the anaesthetist, although there are occasions when we are approached directly by patients for advice about referral.

Finally, the GMC warns that:

If you charge fees, you must tell the patient if part of the fee goes to another doctor.

This is a reference to the practice of 'fee-splitting', whereby a specialist would pay a proportion of the fee to the referring doctor. Consequently, the referral could be seen as being made for financial rather than clinical reasons and, hence, as unethical. Usually, anaesthetists have no opportunity for such practice, but it was commonplace several years ago for general practitioners who also practised as anaesthetists to refer patients to surgeons who they knew would ask them to anaesthetise. Thankfully, this practice is rare these days.

It may be that, like surgeons, an anaesthetist may employ an assistant for major cases and, in such instances, it is quite reasonable to indicate on the invoice to the patient where assistants' fees are charged.

Guidance

A number of documents have been introduced in the past few years laying down guidance and standards in independent health care. In April 1999, the Private Practice Forum of the Academy of Royal Medical Colleges produced Principles for a Private Medicine Quality Framework[4]. The forum, although under the banner of the Academy of Royal Medical Colleges, has representatives from the British Medical Association, the Independent Healthcare Association (representing independent providers), and the Association of British Insurers. The document set out the principles of clinical governance within independent hospital practice, and provided a framework for local guidelines. Guidance is now available from numerous sources, including insurers, private hospital groups and individual medical advisory committees of independent hospitals.

The Care Standards Act (2000)

Perhaps the most far-reaching piece of legislation with regard to the independent health-care sector in recent years is the *Care Standards Act (2000)*. This laid the basis for the regulation of every kind of personal care provision, of which private medical practice is just one element. The National Minimal Standards for independent health care were issued in 2002[5], which cover every conceivable aspect of care, for example, consultant qualifications, children's services, information provision, complaints and risk management. The effect upon clinical practice may be considerable, including scope of practice, involvement in risk management procedures and audit.

There is a section of the standards (Standard A22) that covers anaesthesia, and the scope of these is shown in Box 2.

Box 2: Care Standards Act Minimum Standards for Anaesthesia
The following areas are covered:
• pre-operative assessment
• discussion of possible plans of management with the patient
• information on any drugs or treatments
• development of a care plan
• recording the results of the pre-operative consultation
• consent
• checking equipment and drugs
• confirms the identity of the patient
• presence in the operating theatre throughout the operation
• monitoring and record keeping
• recovery staff
• recovery monitoring
• assessment and relief of pain
• recovery facilities
• criteria for discharge from recovery
• training of recovery staff.

The original intention under the Act was to have a body – the National Care Standards Commission (NCSC) – charged with the task of ensuring that the standards were applied throughout the independent sector. However, following the 2002 budget, it was announced that another body – the Commission for Health Audit and Inspection (CHAI) – would be created in 2003, and that this will take on the responsibilities of the NCSC for inspecting the private health sector.

This shows the detail of regulation now covering our practice. So, from the position, less than ten years ago, when there were no written instructions or defined rules, we are now entering an era when almost every aspect of our professional life is covered by laws, regulations, policies and guidelines.

Relationships

As an anaesthetist, one has relationships with a number of different people or groups of people, and each of these involves different (and sometimes conflicting) ethical considerations.

The patient

It is the patient to whom one owes the primary duty of care, although, of course, it is rare that the patient has made an active choice to select the anaesthetist. The basic tenet is that the standard of care in independent practice must be equal to (not greater or less than) that in the NHS. There are responsibilities on both sides of this arrangement: for the anaesthetist to provide optimum care, and for the patient to pay for that service. There are moves, currently, to develop a code of practice for anaesthetists and their patients in the private health-care sector. Box 3 illustrates an example of such a code, which has been modified from the GMC guidelines[6].

Confidentiality is as important in the private sector as in the NHS. In addition to the traditional ethical duties to the patient, the private medical practitioner now has responsibilities under the *Data Protection Act (1998)*, and will need to consider registration under the provisions of the Act, as, almost inevitably, personal information will be held about patients.

The surgeon

Unless the anaesthetist is part of a group (see below), the relationship with individual surgeons usually becomes the basis for practice. This will commonly be an extension of the relationships engendered within the NHS, and this regular team approach to surgery has many benefits for the patient and other staff involved in their treatment.

It is important, nevertheless, that the anaesthetist maintains his or her independence. Other chapters in this volume stress the importance of anaesthetists retaining their clinical autonomy. The financial aspect of independent health-care adds another dimension to the general ethical considerations in respect of the patient's treatment: one should not compromise one's own standards in the

Box 3: Code of practice for anaesthetists involved in independent practice	
1.	The anaesthetist's overriding responsibility is to the individual patient.
2.	You must be honest in any financial arrangements with patients.
3.	You should provide information about fees and charges before obtaining a patient's consent to treatment.
4.	If you publish information about the services you provide, the information must be factual and verifiable. It must be published in a way that conforms with the law and with the guidance issued by the Advertising Standards Authority.
5.	You must not exploit a patient's vulnerability or lack of medical knowledge when making charges for treatment or services.
6.	If you charge fees, you must tell the patient if any part of the fee goes to any other doctor.
7.	You must be honest in financial and commercial dealings with insurers and individuals.
8.	If you have financial or commercial interests in organisations providing health care, these must not affect the way you prescribe for, treat or refer patients.
9.	The fee for an anaesthetic should include pre- and post-operative care.
10.	Since patients may not have direct contact with anaesthetists before committing themselves to relevant treatment or investigations, anaesthetists should agree their fees with the patient in advance of treatment.
11.	The patient is responsible for payment of the agreed fee. If the patient is insured, they should check with their insurance company whether they will be covered for the whole amount. The insurance company has a responsibility to make it clear to the patient exactly what they will pay for.
12.	Where intensive care unit (ICU) care is usual for the procedure, this should be included in the anaesthetist's fee and agreed with the patient beforehand.
13.	The fee for a single procedure should not be broken down in such a way that charges for individual parts can be made as if they were separate and additional anaesthetics.
14.	Regional procedures may involve prolonged specialist care post-operatively, and fees should be agreed beforehand.

pursuit of income, and neither should one be compromised by the surgeon into undertaking treatment that is not justified.

The relationship between anaesthetist and surgeon may not be so close where the anaesthetist is working in a group practice. Where allocation to a private list has been made by the group's secretary or other mechanism, it is at least good manners to make contact with the surgeon or their secretary beforehand. This will enable exchange of any clinical or administrative information (e.g. fees), which will assist in the patient's treatment.

The insurer

The relationship with the insurer is taking on an increasingly high profile within the independent sector. In 2000, 6.8 million people had private medical insurance. Just under two-thirds of these are insured through company schemes (and, hence, will tend to be healthy), whilst the remainder are individual subscribers. Although the rapid growth of health insurance cover observed during the 1980s has disappeared, fierce competition between insurers is contributing to a growing number of products. Insurers are increasing their profits by raising the cost of premiums and, at the same time, there is a trend towards reducing claims. The increased prices are borne mainly by individual policyholders – between 1990 and 2000 premiums increased by 24% for the corporate market, whilst individual subscribers (who are often more elderly) experienced a 78% rise[7]. The ethical basis of insurance provision can sometimes be seen to be less than ideal, where selling policies to individuals who are unlikely to claim benefits can make the largest profits.

The contract of treatment still lies between the doctor and the patient, but many threats to this are emerging. Direct settlement is the first – whilst seen by the patient as a great convenience, it is removing them from the transaction and giving the impression that it is not their problem. Once again, reliable information on fees pre-operatively should avoid any problems.

Some insurers, notably BUPA, have developed 'partnerships' or other similar arrangements. Here the surgeon or anaesthetist agrees to conform to certain standards, one of which, unsurprisingly, is adherence to a scale of fees. The fact that this has only been taken up by a small minority of anaesthetists speaks for itself.

Some insurers are pursuing even more radical moves, including electronic billing and attempting to break the financial link between the anaesthetist and the patient by making the hospital responsible for reimbursing the anaesthetist. It seems that some insurers would like to control the independent provision of health care, by claiming that they are the champion of the patients needs. However, they cannot get away from the fact that they are driven by the bottom line of the balance sheet.

The National Health Service

Most anaesthetists in the UK who undertake private practice also have contracts with the NHS. Two current developments may affect this: the consultant contract, and revalidation. At present, any consultant employed by the NHS can undertake private practice, albeit with limitations, and most insurers and independent hospitals make an NHS consultant contract a prerequisite for recognition. It was, originally, the stated intention of the government to bar consultants from undertaking independent practice for the first few years, but this has been replaced in the contract agreed with the profession's negotiators by a requirement to do extra work for the NHS. At the time of writing, the contract has yet to be accepted by the profession (and there is considerable opposition to it). However, if it is accepted, it is possible that this may tempt some consultants to forgo an NHS appointment, and work entirely in the private sector, but the second development – revalidation – may make this more difficult, as obtaining the necessary documentation outside the NHS will be difficult and probably expensive. The formation of 'chambers' for consultant practice, as in the legal profession, is another option that is under consideration. It is perhaps the perception that consultants are 'moonlighting' from their NHS contracts to undertake private practice that has created the government's determination, despite repeated surveys showing that, on average, consultants work far longer hours than contracted[8]. Such 'moonlighting' is of course unethical and cause for disciplinary action, but perception of general moonlighting, given the hours consultants actually work for the NHS, is surprising when one considers that the instances of it are actually rare.

The recent developments whereby the NHS is making increased and more imaginative use of the private sector seem to bring additional dilemmas for the consultant. If an operating session that is usually covered by a fixed commitment as part of one's contract is moved to a private facility, it is clear that this is part of one's NHS work. Provided that one has a clear job plan, it is not difficult to identify what work is covered by one's contract and what is additional work.

Should one accept NHS work in the private sector at a lower rate? One of the great advantages of independent work is that this is completely up to the individual, and market forces apply. If one insists on being paid a certain amount for work, it can always be offered to someone else who may well be willing to do it for less money.

Colleagues

The International Code of Medical Ethics reminds us that we should treat our colleagues as we would wish to be treated ourselves, and that we should not entice patients away from them[9]. Independent practice is, by its nature, competitive, but success will rarely follow regular breaches of etiquette. The keys to success have traditionally been cited as the three A's – Ability, Affability and Availability – and it is also generally perceived that these are in the reverse order of importance for a successful practice. This may be true, but availability should not result from relying on one's NHS colleagues (or, worse still, one's trainees) to pick up the pieces.

Several references have already been made to group practices, and where there is such cooperation rather than out-and-out competition between colleagues, this can work not only to their advantage but also to that of the NHS, as members of the group can be more rationally rostered in both sectors. Some groups work just on the basis of such allocation of duties, but it is often where the partnership involves sharing of the financial rewards that there is greatest harmony.

Another advantage of a group practice is the ability to publish a fee scale to provide patients with information on costs of treatment. Working as part of a group practice can ensure that fees are well publicised, but this may then risk prosecution under the *Competition Act (1998)*, which seeks to prevent practices that are anti-competitive.

The decision several years ago by the then Monopolies and Mergers Commission (now replaced by the Competition Commission) to prohibit the British Medical Association from publishing a scale of fees has made it unclear whether any group of anaesthetists can publish a scale. In 1998, a number of insurers jointly commissioned a review of 'relative values' of procedures, and this work was completed in 2000 by Newchurch & Co. None of the insurers have at the time of writing (2002) implemented the scale and, indeed, this scale was referred to the Office of Fair Trading (OFT) during 2001, although it was subsequently ruled that it did not constitute a monopoly. In a more recent development, six group anaesthetic practices are at the time of writing being investigated by the OFT, and it would appear that the basis of this is that the publication of a scale of fees could make them guilty of price-fixing. On the other hand, one insurer is now notably taking a hard line in cases where fees that they consider 'higher than normal' have not been advised to the patient beforehand. Consequently, it would seem that the anaesthetist is caught here between a rock and a hard place over whether to provide adequate information at an appropriate time to the patient.

The outcome of the OFT investigation of anaesthetic practices should, therefore, provide some welcome guidance in this difficult area, but, pending any decision, it would appear that full partnerships based on sharing the income should be in a better position than a loose group of professionals publishing a common scale.

Group practices also solve another practical ethical problem to the independent medical practitioner, that of comprehensive emergency cover. Anaesthetists have a duty to ensure post-operative care for their patients, but this may produce difficulties with availability. Sharing this load amongst a larger number (as in the NHS) can provide a better service for the patients and a better quality of life for the doctor. Indeed, we should not forget ourselves in the list of duties to others! One is unlikely to be able to adhere to the guidelines referred to earlier if one is over-stretched, and 'look after oneself' is never a bad policy.

The hospital

Until relatively recently, the only requirements for undertaking private medical practice of any type was to be on the register of the GMC. Most hospitals, nevertheless, require doctors to apply for the right to practice. The *Care Standards Act (2000)*, referred to above, lays down minimum standards to ensure that patients are treated by appropriately trained and qualified clinicians. Each hospital should now have its own arrangements for implementing clinical governance, and it is the duty of all practitioners to comply with these.

Society

The overriding duty of the anaesthetist is to the individual patient, but there are situations in which an ethical duty is owed to the public at large. Most of these dilemmas are dealt with elsewhere, but it is important to recognise the particular situation in which the anaesthetist finds him or herself in private medical practice. Many high-profile cases of surgical malpractice that have come before the GMC in recent years have involved anaesthetists. In the most widely known case, it was the anaesthetist who first expressed concerns[10] but, in many others, the actions

in NHS hospitals means that individual doctors can treat both their NHS and private patients at the same time in the same place. The arrangement has generated about £300 million per annum for the NHS, but at the cost of opportunities to reduce waiting lists more quickly. As recently as July 2002, the Health Minister thought about reducing the number of paybeds so that NHS patients can use them full time[12]. Although it would not solve all waiting list problems, the reappropriation of paybeds would at least not add to the delays of waiting NHS patients for the sake of NHS income.

Private medicine does not depend on the NHS just through the paybed system. There is the fact that NHS hospitals receive emergency cases from private hospitals which private hospitals are not staffed to cope with (for instance, an unexpected need for immediate intensive care). This means that there is a free public safety net for the private hospitals. The fact that many of the patients in these emergency cases are also entitled to NHS treatment is beside the point: private hospitals are able to keep their costs low by using an unpaid-for safety net underneath them and, where the failure or incompetence of treatment in private hospitals creates the emergency, the NHS is made to pick up the pieces more than financially. When pieces are picked up from the private sector, routine emergencies in the public sector are treated less efficiently.

It might be thought that the dependence of private and public systems of medicine is mutual and extensive enough to make the claim of one-way dependence on the public sector suspect. If it were not for vacant private beds in private hospitals, the NHS would be even more lamentably equipped to cope with seasonal increases in demand for beds than it now is. If it were not for the occasional joint venture between the NHS and private health insurers in capital projects, the public purse would be more heavily burdened than it would otherwise be. There is some truth in this, but the extent to which the private sector in medicine is an *independent* sector is easy to exaggerate. Consider the analogy between the private and public sectors in hospital medicine in the UK, compared with the private and public sectors in education. In private education, as in private hospital medicine, the public pays twice, but there is more of a sense in education than in the hospital sector of medicine of two fully functioning systems, albeit unequal in size. There are the two sets – one public, one private – of school buildings, playing grounds and so on; two sets of staff; two sets of pupils. It is true that that there are private hospital buildings in the UK – over 200 – in addition to public ones. But these are not general hospitals, in the way that private schools are general schools offering the same range of subjects as a state-funded school, or even a wider range. Were private education to be modelled on private hospital medicine, one would have the spectacle of state school teachers spending their spare time in private schools teaching core subjects, or going from state classroom to private classroom within the same state school building; or the same pupils taking some classes in the state school and getting some limited tuition in a private school. The most striking dissimilarity between the private and public sectors in the two areas is the double deployment of staff and facilities in hospitals: staff and facilities that are primarily publicly funded. If the costs of educating doctors are also taken into account, the public subsidy of private medicine is even greater.

There are no private medical schools in the UK. The huge costs of medical education are barely reflected in the fees paid by medical students, if they pay any, but those costs are borne by the public sector in the UK. It is probably true that there are hidden subsidies of the private education system in the UK as well. The charitable status of private schools reduces their costs, and some private schools have become very wealthy, partly through being charities. But I do not say that this subsidy is fairer in private education than in medicine.

Barham does not consider these points. He does speak of the issue of whether doctors in private practice put in the hours they owe to the NHS, and he claims that often they do *more* than they owe. I do not want to dispute this claim. But I want to suggest that the NHS experience of doctors in private practice is beneficial to them and beneficial to private patients in ways that, again, count as a hidden subsidy to the private sector. Barham says that the surgical teams that anaesthetists form in private practice grow out of those that exist in the NHS. He implies that the same teams work together in the NHS and private practice. The continuity of the teams and their shared experience is an asset to the teams themselves and to their NHS patients, but it is a saleable asset in the private sector, with the benefits in that sector going mainly to the doctors and private patients. Of course, the work done in the private sector may be extra work in what is already a very heavy schedule in the NHS, and the doctors doing that extra work deserve to be compensated. The question is: on what basis? Consulting services provided by full-time employees of universities are usually conditional on a hefty overhead being paid to the university. This is justified not only by the university paying for full-time work, but also by the value added to consulting services by activities carried on during paid work in the university. The university deserves its cut because it has enhanced the skills of the consultant. I suggest it is the same for the NHS. It, too, deserves an overhead. Either that, or it can justifiably count on the exclusive use of a new consultant's time for a period of years.

Conflicts of interest

I pass now to an issue raised by Barham's paper for anaesthetists in particular, rather than doctors in general, namely: conflicts of interest. Barham refers with distaste to a practice he thinks has become rare, involving GPs also working as anaesthetists. The practice consists of a GP referring a patient to a particular surgeon in return for an appointment as anaesthetist during the surgery. The danger to impartial referring of this arrangement is obvious. Even if the surgeons and anaesthetists cooperating in such an arrangement are, impersonally speaking, very skilled medical professionals, the possibility of undermining the confidence of patients who came to know of the arrangement is clearly great, so Barham is right to see moral danger in connection with it.

Yet he seems comfortable with other arrangements that are similar. He admits that anaesthetists depend on surgeons for referrals, and yet he does not appear to consider that this might generate a conflict of interest. An anaesthetist who owes a lot of highly paid work to a particular surgeon will probably feel beholden to that surgeon. Perhaps that debt will be called in when the surgeon has made a surgical mistake, in which case an injustice is done to the patient. Or perhaps referrals are expected by a surgeon to be met with tolerance of occasional incompetence or sloppiness. Operating room teams without financial dealings with one another might run a smaller risk of conflict of interest along such lines. This is a consideration in favour of surgical teams as financed within the NHS system, but it is also an argument for arrangements that do not involve occasional financial obligations to people one works with in private practice *as well as* in the NHS. Yet, if one worked with entirely different groups in private and NHS work, the medical benefits of working together will be fewer.

Private insurers

Barham has a number of complaints about private medical insurers. First, the ways in which they classify, and are prepared to pay for, medical procedures is sometimes arbitrary. Second, they can sometimes be unprepared to pay all legitimate charges under a private health policy. Third, their role as funders of treatment sometimes gives the patient a false sense of having no ultimate responsibility to pay for medical treatment. Fourth, insurers sometimes enter into what Barham regards as dubious partnerships with anaesthetists in return for predictable or depressed charges. The fact that few anaesthetists are involved in these partnerships, he says, 'speaks for itself'.

Taking the point about 'partnerships' first, Barham seems to be insinuating a kind of monopolistic collusion between private insurers and certain doctors. But this seems no more sinister than car breakdown services that are subcontracted to particular local car repair businesses, at agreed rates, by national firms. The subcontracting and the agreed rates, admittedly, keep costs to the national car breakdown service lower, just as the agreed fees keep costs down to insurers, but this is beneficial, on balance, if premiums are lower as a result and affordable enough for many people to have the chance of quicker treatment. (For the general benefits of private medical insurance in the UK context see Cavers[13].) The agreed fees and the partnerships are, in any case, no harder to justify in private medical insurance than they are in the house insurance market, where they act against cowboy tradesmen who exploit the ignorance of ordinary people about plumbing, wiring and structural repairs.

'Partnership' arrangements benefit insurers, but they may also benefit anaesthetists and other private practitioners, by making bills predictable and avoiding disputes and litigation in relation to charges. An anaesthetist who receives both a lower fee promptly and plenty of repeat business may have better cash flow and less stress than someone who deals outside a partnership with slow-paying and quarrelsome clients who nevertheless 'agree' in the first place to higher fees.

Barham has a good point, however, about the way in which direct payments from insurers insulate patients from a sense of their obligation to settle the charges for private treatment. It can do no harm for patients always to know how much the procedure costs, even if someone else is paying, and, in other areas of insurance, the insurance policy-holder is the one who contracts with tradesmen to do work carried out under the policy, and knows what the tender prices are, even though it is the insurers or their agents who have put out the tenders, who monitor the work, and who pay.

References

1. Gauntlett I. A patient who changed my practice. Royal Coll Anaesthetists Bull 2000; 7: 323–4
2. Weller R. Ethical Issues in Anaesthesia. In: Ethical Issues in Anaesthesia. WE Scott, MD Vickers, H Draper, eds. Butterworth-Heinemann, 1994: 177–85
3. General Medical Council. Good Medical Practice. London: GMC, 1998 [www.gmc-uk.org]
4. Academy of Royal Medical Colleges (Private Practice Forum). Principles for a Private Medicine Quality Framework, 1999 [www.aomrc.org.uk]
5. Department of Health. Independent Healthcare National Minimal Standards Regulations, 2002 [www.doh.gov.uk/ncsc/independenthealthcareregs.pdf]
6. J Wedley – personal communication
7. Laing & Buisson PMI Market Sector Report, 2001 [www.laingbuisson.co.uk/statistics/pmimain.html]
8. British Medical Association – Consultant Contract Roadshow (www.bma.org.uk)
9. World Medical Association International Code of Medical Ethics [www.wma.net/e/policy/17-a_e.html]
10. Learning from Bristol: the report of the public inquiry into children's heart surgery at the Bristol Royal Infirmary 1984–1995. Command Paper: CM 5207
11. Brown S. Private health care: the issue explained. 2001 Guardian [http://society.guardian.c.uk/privatehealthcare/story/0,8150,459397,00.html]
12. Sparrow, A. Milburn wants to end pay beds. Daily Telegraph 15 July 2002 [http://www.dailytelegraph.co.uk/news/2002/07/15/npaybdis.xml]
13. Cavers, D. More private health insurance is desirable and inevitable. In: Health Care, Ethics, and Insurance. T Sorell, ed. Routledge, 1998: 151–64

Index